Understanding your

EYES: CATARACTS, GLAUCOMA & MACULAR DEGENERATION

Mr Robert Walters

Published by Family Doctor Publications Limited
in association with the British Medical Association

IMPORTANT NOTICE

This book is intended not as a substitute for personal medical advice but as a supplement to that advice for the patient who wishes to understand more about his or her condition.

Before taking any form of treatment YOU SHOULD ALWAYS CONSULT YOUR MEDICAL PRACTITIONER.

In particular (without limit) you should note that advances in medical science occur rapidly and some of the information about drugs and treatment contained in this booklet may very soon be out of date.

Family Doctor Publications, PO Box 4664, Poole, Dorset BH15 1NN

Medical Editor: Dr Tony Smith
Consultant Editors: Victoria Gilbert & Mary Fox
Cover Artist: Dave Eastbury
Medical Artist: Peter Cox Associates
Design: MPG Design, Blandford Forum, Dorset
Printing: Reflex Litho, Thetford, Norfolk, using acid-free paper

ISBN: 1 903474 01 9

Contents

Introduction

As you get older, it's natural for your eyesight to deteriorate slightly and for you to need reading spectacles (glasses) or stronger distance glasses. However, there are also some specific eye conditions that can affect older people and it is important for you to be aware of these. Cataracts, glaucoma and macular degeneration are the most common causes of poor vision in the United Kingdom. Each predominantly affects people of middle age and beyond.

Many people with visual difficulties in later life are unnecessarily frightened that they are going to experience progressive visual loss that will curtail their lifestyle or threaten their independence. This book is designed to provide you with comprehensive and simple explanations of common eye conditions and of their causes and treatments. It is intended to supplement information and advice given to you by your general practitioner (GP), optometrist (optician) and hospital eye specialist (ophthalmologist). If you are concerned that you have an eye problem, you should seek professional help.

CATARACTS

Cataracts (clouding of the lenses of the eyes – see page 24) are estimated to affect over a million people in the UK and cataract surgery is by far the most common operation performed in British eye units, with about 150,000 operations every year. Cataract surgery has been carried out for thousands of years and it is known that the ancient Egyptians commonly performed operations for mature cataracts by couching. Couching involves introducing a sharp implement, such as a thorn, into the eye in order to dislocate a mature cataractous lens away from the visual axis or to pierce it so that it mostly reabsorbs. This procedure remained the principal form of treatment for cataracts until the late nineteenth century.

Over the last 50 years, astonishing advances have been made, the most notable of which has been the introduction of a procedure (intraocular lens implantation), which permanently replaces the cataractous lens removed from the eye during cataract surgery with a synthetic lens implant. Patients no longer need to wear the thick, heavy spectacles that were previously necessary after cataract surgery. Indeed, after their operation, many people do not need any spectacles for everyday distance vision.

The pioneering work with intraocular lens implantation was carried out by a British eye surgeon, Mr Harold Ridley, in London in 1949 using shaped Perspex. This remarkable advance followed observation of RAF pilots during World War II who had had perforating eye injuries from the shattered Perspex canopies of their planes.

Mr Ridley noted that the Perspex inside the eye was inert and did not cause any inflammation, and reasoned that Perspex could be made into a lens shape and implanted in the eye to restore the sight of those whose natural lens had been removed because of a cataract. Perspex intraocular lens implants are still used today all over the world, although other materials, such as acrylic, are also utilised. Harold Ridley was knighted, in recognition of his contribution, in 1999 shortly before he died.

Until the late 1970s, everyone undergoing cataract surgery had to stay in hospital for five days or longer. The surgery carried such great risks that it was considered only if the cataract was causing severe visual loss. These days, technical innovations such as microscopic surgery, advanced materials and instrument design, and surgery using small incisions mean that most cataract operations are carried out as day-case procedures and the chances of success are very high. People no longer have to wait until their vision is severely impaired to have a cataract operation but can proceed to surgery when their symptoms are beginning to affect aspects of their everyday life, such as driving or reading.

GLAUCOMA

Glaucoma (see page 49) is a term that covers a variety of conditions characterised by high pressure within the eye and a gradual loss of the peripheral (side) field of vision. It is estimated that there are 300,000 people in the UK with varying degrees of glaucoma, although most forms do not occur until after the age of 40 years and have no symptoms until the late stages. Most optometrists in the UK carry out a comprehensive screening programme for glaucoma. If you are over the age of 40, your optometrist will measure your eye pressure using a simple procedure during a routine eye test. If your eye pressure is higher than normal, your optometrist can refer you to your GP to be considered for a consultation with a hospital eye specialist. The condition can be treated and, if it is diagnosed early on, there is a good chance of preventing serious visual loss.

MACULAR DEGENERATION

Macular degeneration (see page 69) usually only affects people older than 60 years, and thus is known as 'age-related' macular degeneration. There are other forms of the disease that affect younger people, but these are rare and beyond the scope of this book. Macular degeneration can cause difficulties with your central (reading) vision as a result of changes in the most sensitive part of your retina which is called the macula.

Age-related macular degener-ation is surprisingly common; it is estimated that 10 per cent of people aged between 65 and 75 are affected to some degree, rising to 30 per cent of those older than 75. Wearing stronger spectacles and using other visual aids can help many of those with the disease. Even in the worst form of the disease, where the central vision is severely impaired, the peripheral (side) vision is not usually affected so that navigation around the home and out and about is still possible. People who have age-related macular degeneration gain great comfort from the knowledge that they will never go blind or lose their sight completely from this condition.

Although cataracts, glaucoma and macular degeneration are not interrelated they can coexist because they are all conditions that affect people as they get older. If you have macular degeneration and cataracts, then removal of the cataracts can still lead to an improvement in vision although the degree of improvement depends on the severity of the macular degener-ative changes and the cataract. Usually the cataractous lens has to be significantly interfering with the vision before removal would be recommended in patients with severe macular degeneration, but a consultation with and examination by the hospital eye specialist (ophthalmologist) will allow you to

1. OPHTHALMOLOGIST (OPHTHALMIC SURGEON)

An ophthalmologist is a qualified doctor of medicine who has undergone considerable further postgraduate hospital training in the diagnosis and treatment (both medical and surgical) of eye disease. This comprehensive training takes approximately 10 years after obtaining the basic medical degree and all hospital consultants will have obtained specialist postgraduate qualifications including a Fellowship of the Royal College of Ophthalmologists in the UK or its equivalent from Scotland or overseas.

Many of the older ophthalmologists will also have qualified as fellows of the Royal College of Surgeons of England, Edinburgh or Glasgow as this was the usual qualification obtained before the formation of the College of Ophthalmologists (later given the 'Royal' prefix) in 1986.

Within the hospital structure the leading ophthalmologists are the consultants. When visiting the hospital eye department you will not always be seen by a consultant ophthalmologist but may be seen by one of the other staff. These are divided into the training grade staff who are training to become consultant ophthalmologists and non-consultant ophthalmic medical staff.

The training grades are divided into senior house officers – SHOs (undergoing basic surgical training) – and specialist registrars – SPRs (undergoing higher surgical training). The other doctors commonly found in hospital eye departments are the non-consultant grades and these consist of clinical assistants, staff grade doctors and associate specialists. All non-consultant grade doctors will have completed some specialist training in ophthalmology and many will have obtained specialist qualifications from the Royal College of Ophthalmologists or its equivalent. They have not, however, been appointed as consultant ophthalmologists.

All non-consultant and training grade doctors are under the supervision of the consultants who carry the ultimate clinical responsibility for patients under their care. The hospital eye service is usually provided by a combination of consultants, doctors undergoing postgraduate training and non-consultant grades often in association with nurse practitioners and occasionally optometrists.

2. OPTOMETRIST

This term was introduced in the 1980s to distinguish between more highly qualified opticians and dispensing opticians (see below). An optometrist has obtained a professional degree in optometry and is trained in refraction, dispensing of spectacles and basic eye diseases. They do not carry out surgery or prescribe medications other than simple eye lubricants. The College of Optometrists is the professional body representing them in the UK. The regulatory and disciplinary body of optometrists (and dispensing opticians) is the General Optical Council of the UK. There are approximately 11,000 optometrists in the UK.

3. DISPENSING OPTICIAN

A dispensing optician is qualified to dispense spectacles but not to carry out the refraction necessary to determine the power of the lenses within the spectacles. Dispensing opticians are thus not as highly qualified as optometrists but make a significant contribution to optometric practice. There are approximately 8,600 dispensing opticians in the UK.

4. NURSE PRACTITIONERS

Increasing numbers of specially qualified higher grade nurses are found in hospital eye departments in the UK. These are termed 'nurse practitioners' and usually have a specialist nursing qualification in ophthalmology (Diploma in Ophthalmic Nursing). These specialist nurses make up an important part of the ophthalmic service and have many roles. For example, ophthalmic casualty nurses treat simple eye conditions such as corneal abrasions, glaucoma nurses measure intraocular pressures and carry out field tests, and treatment nurses are involved in minor operations such as removing lid cysts.

5. ORTHOPTISTS

Orthoptists are one of the professions allied to medicine (PAMs) and are professionally qualified in the study and treatment of eye movement conditions such as squints. Although this makes up the bulk of their work, in many departments they also carry out glaucoma screening, visual field testing and sometimes ophthalmic photography. There are approximately 1,000 qualified orthoptists in the UK.

receive definitive advice. Your optometrist may also be able to help with advice on this issue.

Glaucoma and macular degeneration, although not strictly interrelated, are both more common in people who are short-sighted (myopes) and therefore it is particularly important that people who are short-sighted should visit their optometrists every one to two years for a check-up.

KEY POINTS

✓ Cataracts are common in elderly people but vision can easily be restored with cataract surgery, which nowadays is a straightforward and safe procedure

✓ Glaucoma is a silent condition which causes a gradual loss of peripheral vision. Your optometrist/optician will screen you for glaucoma when you have an eye test so that sight-saving treatment can be commenced early

✓ Macular degeneration causes central or visual loss but never causes blindness

Your eyes and how they work

Your eyes are among the most highly specialised and sensitive organs of your body. The eye, optic nerve and brain work together to produce an image. To enable you to see, light rays must pass through your cornea, pupil and lens to be focused on your retina (see figure on page 8). An electrical signal is generated in the retina and passed along the optic nerve to specialist parts of the brain where the image is interpreted. Vision is truly the king of all the senses.

THE EYELIDS, ORBIT AND TEAR FILM

Your eyes are protected by bony eye sockets (the orbits) and are cushioned by a layer of fat. Your eyelids provide thick protective coats with lashes that help to prevent foreign bodies such as dirt and dust entering your eye. They also spread a special liquid (tears) over the surface of your eyes at regular intervals. The tear film is produced by the lacrimal gland, which lies slightly above your eyeball in the outer upper part of your eye socket. Tears prevent the eyes from drying out and protect them from infections. The tears are spread by the blinking action of your eyelids and drain away into two canals (tear ducts) at the inner part of your eyelids and then through a fine tube to your nose.

We only notice tears when excess liquid is produced, for example, when we cry. The tears drain away through your nose and this is one reason why crying can block your nose. If the tears are reduced in volume or the quality of the tear film is poor the eyes feel dry and uncomfortable. A large variety of artificial tears is available at the chemist which can soothe dry eyes but can never completely replace the natural tear film.

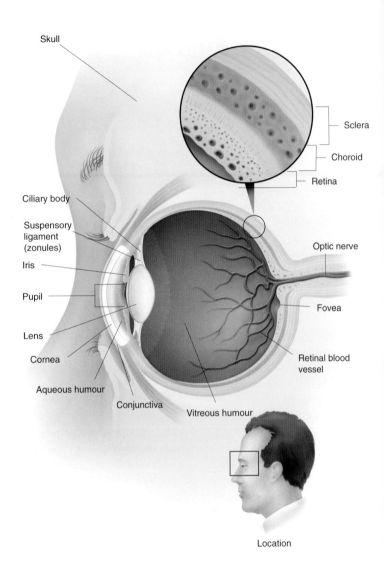

Skull

Sclera

Choroid

Retina

Ciliary body

Suspensory
ligament
(zonules)

Iris

Pupil

Lens

Cornea

Aqueous humour

Conjunctiva

Vitreous humour

Optic nerve

Fovea

Retinal blood
vessel

Location

This illustration shows the principal features of the eye. The eyeball is protected by the
bony eye socket and cushioned by a layer of fat. Each eyeball is roughly spherical.

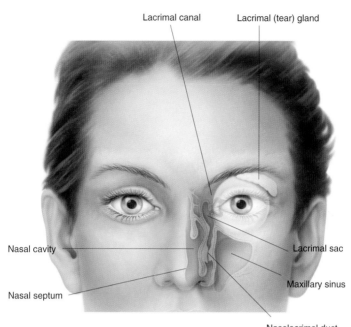

Lacrimal canal

Lacrimal (tear) gland

Nasal cavity

Lacrimal sac

Maxillary sinus

Nasal septum

Nasolacrimal duct

Tears are produced by the lacrimal gland. Tears prevent the eyes from drying out and protect them from infection. Tears drain away through the nose.

EYE MOVEMENTS

Your eyes swivel in their sockets using six delicate muscles attached to the outside of each eye. These muscles control the position of the eyes so accurately that, when you are reading a book, they can pinpoint successive lines of text in less than one hundredth of a second. The movement of your eye muscles is controlled by three nerves that come directly from your brain (the third, fourth and sixth cranial nerves). The front surface of the eye has a clear central portion (the cornea) and the rest is covered by a waterproof protective layer (the conjunctiva) which extends from the edges of the cornea to cover around one-third of the eyeball. Beneath the conjunctiva lies the sclera, a tough fibrous layer that provides the main structural wall of your eyeball. The sclera and conjunctiva form the 'white of your eye'.

INSIDE YOUR EYES

The cornea is the clear central portion of the front of your eye. It is

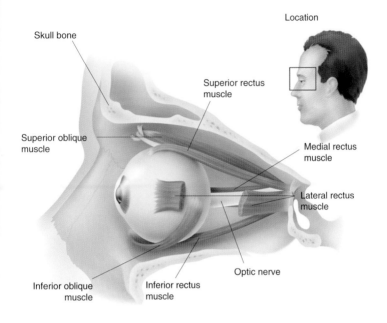

Location

Skull bone

Superior rectus muscle

Superior oblique muscle

Medial rectus muscle

Lateral rectus muscle

Inferior oblique muscle

Inferior rectus muscle

Optic nerve

Each eye swivels in the eye socket using six delicate and very precise muscles attached to the outside of the eyeball.

strong and allows light to pass through it. The cornea carries out most of the focusing of the eye. It refracts (bends) light entering your eye onto the lens behind the pupil, which then fine-tunes the focusing of the image so that it falls accurately on the retina at the back of the eye. The iris – the coloured tissue around the pupil – is made up of fine layers of muscle with the pupil as a central hole. The pupil is highly sensitive to light, dilating in darkness, or when you are excited, to allow more light into the eye, but quickly constricting for protection if the eye is in bright light. The size of your pupil is controlled by the muscles of the iris. Belladonna eye drops (derived from the deadly nightshade plant and now called atropine) were used by ladies in the court of Louis XIV of France to dilate (widen) their pupils because they believed that it made them look more beautiful. Hence the name 'Bella Donna' which means 'beautiful lady'. The colour of the iris, which determines the colour of your eyes, is inherited from your parents or grandparents.

The eye is made up of two fluid-

Location

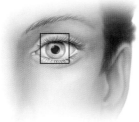

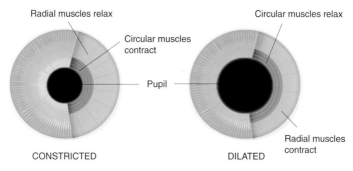

Radial muscles relax

Circular muscles contract

Circular muscles relax

Pupil

Radial muscles contract

CONSTRICTED   DILATED

The iris is made up of fine layers of coloured muscle with the pupil as the central hole. The size of the pupil is controlled by the muscles of the iris in response to the amount of light.

filled chambers. The front chamber, between the lens and the cornea, is filled with a liquid called aqueous humour which bathes and nourishes this part of your eye. The fluid circulates continually. It is produced in the region behind the iris by the ciliary body. The fluid passes around the inside of the eye and through the pupil to leave the eye mainly through a drainage angle called the trabecular meshwork, which lies between the base of the iris and the cornea.

The lens lies behind the pupil and is suspended by a series of very fine threads (the zonules). These threads can tighten or loosen, under the control of a muscle (ciliary muscle) to which they are attached, enabling the lens to become fatter or slimmer. The muscle is circular and shaped like a tyre inner tube with the zonules attached to the inside surface, so when the muscle contracts the size of the circle becomes smaller and the zonules relax. The zonules are in turn attached to the lens of the eye holding the lens in tension so that when the zonules relax the lens can also relax and become fatter in shape increasing the focusing power of the lens. This process is called 'accommodation' and enables the eye to vary its focus from a distant object to one that is closer. Thus, for looking at near objects (such as reading a book) the 'ciliary muscle' as it is called contracts and allows the lens to become fatter, therefore bending the light rays more and focusing the image on the retina. Conversely, for viewing objects in the distance the ciliary muscle will relax thereby tightening the zonules and stretching the lens, which will then bend the light rays less and focus the light once again on the retina.

This process is demonstrated in the figure below.

The lens in the eye is translucent and has no direct blood supply as it derives the nutrients and oxygen it requires from the fluid in which it is bathed (the aqueous humour). Clouding or opacities within the lens are termed cataracts and these are discussed in more detail in the chapter on page 24. The lens is shaped like a Smartie sweet and has an outer 'capsule' and an inner 'nucleus' and 'cortex'.

The second fluid-filled chamber lies behind the lens. It is large and filled with a clear jelly-like substance called the 'vitreous humour'. This is

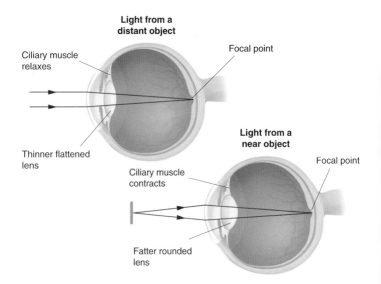

Light from a distant object

Focal point

Ciliary muscle relaxes

Thinner flattened lens

Light from a near object

Focal point

Ciliary muscle contracts

Fatter rounded lens

Accommodation is the process by which the eye can vary its focus from a distant object to a close object.

important in the formation of your eye in the uterus (particularly the lens) but has no known significant function after birth. In middle age and beyond the vitreous humour tends to shrink down and lose some of its clarity, forming 'floaters' which are commonly noticed in the vision particularly in bright light looking at a plain light-coloured surface. The vitreous humour does not circulate like the aqueous humour which passes around the outside of it.

The retina lines the inside of the back of the eye. It is a wafer-thin layer containing light-sensitive cells called photoreceptors (rods and cones). There are about 130 million photoreceptors in each eye.

The rod photoreceptors (about 123 million) lie in the peripheral (outer) part of the retina and deal with black and white vision. The rods are sensitive to low-intensity light, but cannot differentiate between colours, which is why objects appear to lose colour at night.

Colour vision is served by the cone photoreceptors, which are fewer in number (about seven million) and work best in high-intensity light. There are three types of cones; each type responds to a different primary colour (red, blue and green). Cones are concentrated in the centre of the retina (the macula). The macula specialises in detailed vision, such as that used for reading and recognising faces.

Some people are born with mild defects in one or more of the three kinds of cones and this leads to colour blindness. For example, eight per cent of men are red/green colour blind, being unable to distinguish clearly between red and green. This can mean that they cannot clearly tell the difference between a red and green traffic light, but can drive safely because they know that the top light means stop and the bottom light means go.

Nerve fibres connect the photoreceptors to the brain. The millions of nerve connections from the retina collect together in the optic nerve; there are two optic nerves, one for each of the eyes. At the base of the brain, the two optic nerves join and then divide into separate channels (tracts). After further processing, the nerves pass to the occipital cortex, a specialist part of the brain at the back of the head that interprets the visual signals as images.

HOW YOU SEE

The visual system can be likened to two video cameras (your eyes) connected to a computer (your brain) by connecting electrical cables (the optic nerves). The cornea and lens form the focusing mechanism of the camera. They focus light to form an image that is

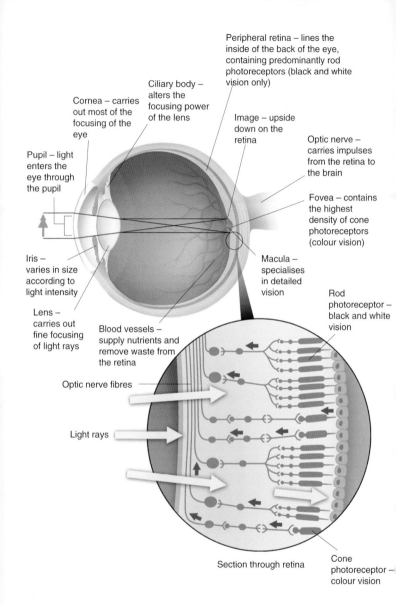

The function of the components of the eye in vision.

Cornea – carries out most of the focusing of the eye

Ciliary body – alters the focusing power of the lens

Peripheral retina – lines the inside of the back of the eye, containing predominantly rod photoreceptors (black and white vision only)

Image – upside down on the retina

Optic nerve – carries impulses from the retina to the brain

Pupil – light enters the eye through the pupil

Fovea – contains the highest density of cone photoreceptors (colour vision)

Iris – varies in size according to light intensity

Macula – specialises in detailed vision

Lens – carries out fine focusing of light rays

Blood vessels – supply nutrients and remove waste from the retina

Rod photoreceptor – black and white vision

Optic nerve fibres

Light rays

Section through retina

Cone photoreceptor – colour vision

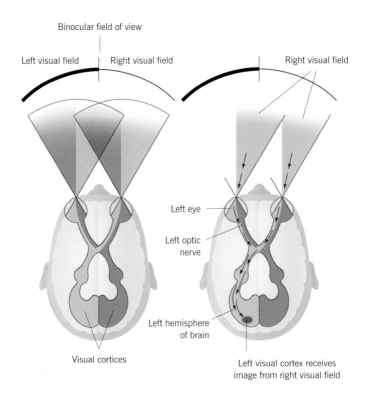

Binocular field of view

Left visual field | Right visual field

Right visual field

Left eye

Left optic nerve

Left hemisphere of brain

Visual cortices

Left visual cortex receives image from right visual field

The left side of the brain processes images from the right visual field (in both eyes) and vice versa.

projected onto the retina at the back of the eye. The photoreceptors in the retina then translate the light energy into an electrical signal, which is transmitted along the optic nerves to a specialist part of the brain (the visual cortices). The picture on the retina is upside down and back to front. However, your brain learns and becomes pro-grammed from birth to interpret this image the right way up. The visual cortices interpret the electrical signals received from your eyes and translate these into the image that you see in your mind. This immense-ly complicated process is only partially understood.

Sight is such an important sense that a large proportion of the brain is dedicated to interpreting what you see. Interestingly, the left side of your brain deals with images from your right visual field (in both eyes) and the right side of your brain with images from your left visual field. Therefore, people who have a stroke affecting the visual cortex on one side of their brain find that the opposite half of their visual field is blanked out in both eyes.

KEY POINTS

✓ Your eyes are highly specialised complicated organs

✓ Each eye works like a camera: light rays pass through your pupil and are focused by your lens and cornea on to your retina

✓ Your retina contains millions of light-sensitive cells

Common sight problems

In some people, the image is not naturally focused on the retina, and these people are said to be short-sighted (myopic) or long-sighted (hypermetropic). Other people may see a distorted image as a result of astigmatism. These common sight problems can be readily diagnosed during routine eye tests and can usually be corrected with spectacles (glasses) or contact lenses. Ageing can also affect your eyes, making it more difficult for you to see close up (a sight problem called 'presbyopia').

EYE TESTS

It is important to have regular eye examinations as part of your normal health regimen so that your eyes can be examined internally and externally. This is a simple and painless procedure involving the testing of your visual acuity, examination of the eye with a microscope and a measurement of the intraocular pressure. An eye examination typically takes 20 to 30 minutes and is usually combined with a refraction test (testing for glasses) by your optometrist. The eye movements and coordination will also be assessed. If the vision is becoming blurred because of refractive errors (see below), then these can be simply corrected with a pair of spectacles supplied by the optometrist. If the examination by the optometrist gives rise to a suspicion of eye disease (such as cataracts or glaucoma), then the optometrist will refer you to a hospital eye specialist (ophthalmologist). This referral is usually coordinated with your general practitioner. The vision is measured using a standardised lit chart (a Snellen chart). This test is always carried out at a standard distance of six metres (albeit sometimes using a mirror). This is illustrated in the figure on page 19. If you have normal vision you should be able to read the standard six-metre line at six metres away and your visual acuity would then be described as 6/6. If your vision is reduced, you may only be able to read the larger letters above the six-metre line, for example, those that a person with 'normal vision' would be able to read at a distance of nine metres away. Your visual acuity would then be described as 6/9. Similarly if you were only able to read the top letter on the chart six metres away which someone with normal vision should be able to read 60 metres away, your visual acuity would be described as 6/60 and would be poor. The metric system is used in the vast majority of countries throughout the world but in North America they have persisted in the use of feet rather than metres and therefore normal visual acuity of 6/6 in the UK would be described as 20/20 in North America. Snellen chart vision testing is an extremely helpful standard method which is used throughout the world but does not take into account other aspects of visual function, for example, contrast sensitivity and glare. If necessary more complex measurements can be carried out in specialist eye departments.

As well as eye diseases, signs of other health problems such as high blood pressure and diabetes can be picked up at a routine eye test as they can show changes in the retina. If detected early enough, these conditions can be treated and managed effectively before complications such as sight loss can develop. It is therefore a sensible precaution to have an eye examination at least every two years. All eye examinations by the optician/optometrist for people aged 60 and over and 18 or under are free of charge. Free eye tests are also available on the NHS to other groups of people, including those with diabetes and glaucoma, people aged 40 and over who are the parent/brother/sister/child of someone with glaucoma, and those who are blind or partially sighted.

Refraction (testing for glasses) is painless and straightforward and usually involves a two-stage process. The first is an objective test, the refractionist using a 'retinoscope' to shine a slit-shaped beam of light into the eye and putting up corrective lenses in front of the eye until the refractive error is neutralised. This is followed by a subjective test in which the lenses are put up into a trial frame in front of the eyes and small changes are made to the lenses while asking the patient whether the vision is better or worse with those changes. The initial refraction is carried out for distance vision and then different lenses are used for testing near vision until both distance vision and

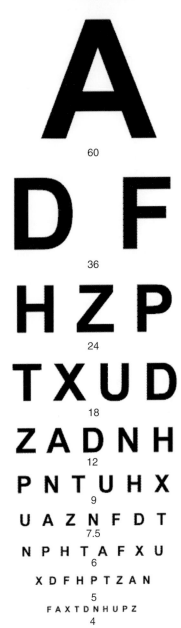

A

60

D F

36

H Z P

24

T X U D

18

Z A D N H

12

P N T U H X

9

U A Z N F D T

7.5

N P H T A F X U

6

X D F H P T Z A N

5

F A X T D N H U P Z

4

Snellen chart – the chart shown is for illustration only and is of no use for eye testing.

near vision are clear with the appropriate lenses. These are then prescribed for your glasses. If you require spectacles for distance vision only then distance glasses alone will be supplied. If you require spectacles to correct your vision for both near and distance then bifocal lenses can be supplied or separate reading and distance glasses, according to individual needs and requirements. Varifocal lenses are also available. These consist of graded lenses which allow people to see in the distance through the top part of the lens, which then become progressively more powerful in the lower portions of the lens in order to facilitate clear vision at middle distances and for near vision also. These Varifocal lenses have become more sophisticated recently and are increasingly popular. Trifocal lenses are relatively rare nowadays and consist of a three-part lens within the spectacle, one for distance, one for middle distance and one for near. They have largely been replaced by Varifocal lenses.

An optometrist will be able to check your vision, prescribe glasses if necessary and carry out a routine screening of your eyes as detailed above. Your general practitioner would also be able to give you a simple examination of your eyes, visual system and eye movements if disease is suspected. Many general practice groups have specialist GPs who have added training in monitoring conditions such as diabetes and will have added expertise in examining the retina for the signs of this disease. If eye disease is suspected or has been found, then a referral to a consultant ophthalmologist within the hospital eye service would be made. Specialist medical eye training in Britain is sophisticated and carried out to the highest standard. You can be confident that the hospital eye department will be well equipped and staffed by doctors, nurses and other staff who have been well trained. Many of the bigger hospital eye departments in the UK now contain supra-specialist eye consultants who, in addition to a general knowledge of eye conditions and treatments, will have a specialist interest in a certain branch of ophthalmology such as eye movement disorders (squints), glaucoma, retinal disease, oculoplastic disorders and many others.

REFRACTIVE ERRORS

Long-sightedness (hypermetropia)

If you are long-sighted, seeing close up may take more effort and can trigger headaches and blurred vision. In long-sightedness the image of a nearby object is formed behind your retina, rather than on it.

This is either because your eyeball is too short or occasionally because your cornea is not curved enough. The majority of people are born mildly long-sighted but do not require spectacles as they can focus through their long-sightedness which gradually reduces in the first 10 years of life. People who are very long-sighted require spectacles from childhood, although the power of these may reduce during their teenage years before levelling off. People who are long-sighted in childhood require glasses for reading at an earlier age than normal. Long-sightedness can be corrected with spectacles or contact lenses using a lens that refracts (bends) the light more (a positive

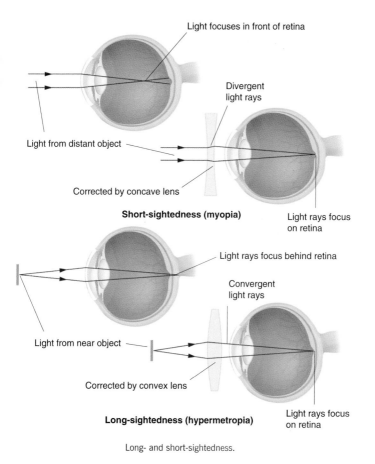

Long- and short-sightedness.

powered convex lens) so that it focuses accurately on your retina.

Short-sightedness (myopia)

If you are short-sighted, the opposite applies. You can see nearby objects easily, but looking at distant objects (for example, road signs) is more difficult. In short-sightedness the light from a distant object is focused in front of your retina. This is because either your eyeball is too long or less frequently because your cornea is too curved. Short-sightedness usually develops in childhood (before the age of 20 years) and tends to stabilise in adulthood. It can be corrected by wearing spectacles or contact lenses, using a 'negative' powered concave lens to achieve accurate focusing of the image on your retina.

People who are short-sighted often do not require reading glasses in later years (unlike the rest of the population) because they find that they can read by taking their glasses off. Some people, however, prefer to have bifocal or Varifocal lenses so that they do not have to remove their spectacles to read.

Astigmatism

If you have astigmatism, your cornea may be curved more in one direction than the other (shaped more like a rugby ball rather than a football) or your lens may bend the light unequally. You may notice that objects are blurred or out of focus. Astigmatism is usually inherited and may be present at birth, although it may develop from a corneal scar or from surgery (for example, for cataracts). Spectacles or contact lenses can be made to correct this focusing abnormality.

Laser surgery for refractive errors

Detailed discussion about this topic is beyond the scope of this book but there has been increasing interest in laser surgery for the correction of a variety of refractive errors. Relatively low degrees of short-sightedness (up to six dioptres) can be accurately corrected with laser treatment and recent advances have also led to successful correction of low degrees of long-sightedness and astigmatism. However, it should be borne in mind that all of these refractive errors can be corrected with spectacles or contact lenses and that laser treatment is a form of surgery and carries a small risk of damage to the eyes. It is recommended that anyone contemplating laser treatment for refractive error should seek advice from an ophthalmologist or optometrist before making any decisions. Information is available from the Royal College of Ophthalmologists at the address in the back of this book.

When cataract surgery is performed short-sightedness and long-sightedness can be corrected by the use of a tailor-made lens implant in the eye. This should be discussed with the consultant ophthalmologist before cataract surgery.

AGEING AND YOUR EYES

As you get older, the lenses in your eyes may lose flexibility and you may find that it gradually becomes more difficult to focus on close objects. Many people notice their near sight deteriorating from around 40 years of age. This is called 'presbyopia' and is a natural part of ageing. It is not a disease and cannot be prevented. However, it is easily corrected with reading glasses.

KEY POINTS

✓ It is important to have regular eye examinations to assess your sight and check for other health problems such as high blood pressure or diabetes

✓ If you are long-sighted, you cannot see close-up objects very clearly; if you are short-sighted, the opposite applies

✓ In astigmatism, your cornea is warped and objects seem blurred

✓ As you get older, your lenses lose flexibility, causing presbyopia

Cataracts

If you have been told by your doctor or optometrist that you have a cataract, you are not alone. Cataracts affect over half of all people aged over 65, they are often slow growing and may take many months or years to affect your vision significantly. Almost all cases of cataract can be treated success-fully and modern cataract surgery is a relatively simple process, often requiring only one day in hospital.

WHAT IS A CATARACT?

Normally, the lens in the eye, which lies behind the pupil, is clear or transparent. It helps to focus light rays on to your retina at the back of the eye. If you have a cataract, however, your lens is cloudy (opaque) to varying degrees. This stops enough light from reaching your retina and the resulting picture is dull and fuzzy.

CAUSES OF CATARACTS

Cataracts have many different causes, including the following.

Developmental problems

A few people are born with cataracts and these are called 'congenital cataracts'. Congenital cataracts may be caused by disease during pregnancy, such as an infection, for example German measles (rubella). Fortunately, such cataracts are rare in the UK, although when they do occur they can sometimes substantially interfere with a baby's vision. If a baby is born with significant cataracts, he or she can be successfully operated upon in a similar way to adults with cataracts but the resulting vision is not always good. All babies in the UK are screened for congenital cataracts which may show up as a white pupil or poor 'red reflex' in the pupil.

Many congenital cataracts are mild and inherited (rather than being related to a disease or infection), and consist of blue or white dots scattered throughout the lens. This type of congenital cataract seldom interferes with the normal development of vision in childhood and usually remains unchanged throughout life.

Age

By far the most common cause of cataracts in the Western World is the ageing process and, if we live long enough, most of us will develop cataracts to some extent. As you get older, changes occur in the proteins in the lens, causing it to harden and lose elasticity. The proteins may also clump together and form a cataract.

Trauma

Trauma, such as a blow to the eye or a more severe eye injury, intense heat or chemical burns, can damage the lens of your eye, leading to the development of a cataract. This can occur at any age.

Other causes

Some diseases such as diabetes mellitus (both the insulin-dependent and tablet/diet-controlled varieties) can cause significant lens opacities, although these usually occur later in life and after the diabetes has been present for many years. Some drugs (particularly corticosteroids) used for a considerable period of time can also cause cataracts. There is no set pattern for the development of these cataracts but, in general the higher the dose the greater the likelihood of cataract development. Other factors that have been implicated in the development of cataracts include long-standing inflammation in the eye (uveitis or iritis) and ionising radiation such as radiation from nuclear fission or X-rays. Cataracts are also associated with poor levels of nutrition particularly in developing countries but this is not a significant factor in the Western World.

Long-term exposure to high levels of sunshine (particularly ultraviolet light) and smoking have also been cited as causes. However, these last two factors remain controversial.

TYPES OF CATARACT

There are many different forms of cataract, but there are three types that commonly occur as part of the ageing process. Sometimes people may have more than one form.

Nuclear sclerotic cataracts

Nuclear sclerotic cataracts result in the clouding of the central 'nucleus' of the lens. These cataracts are initially yellowish in colour and gradually become browner as they mature. They can uniformly cut out the light, causing blurring of the vision and making colours appear much duller than they really are. They usually take years to affect the vision significantly. This gradual deterioration often causes people

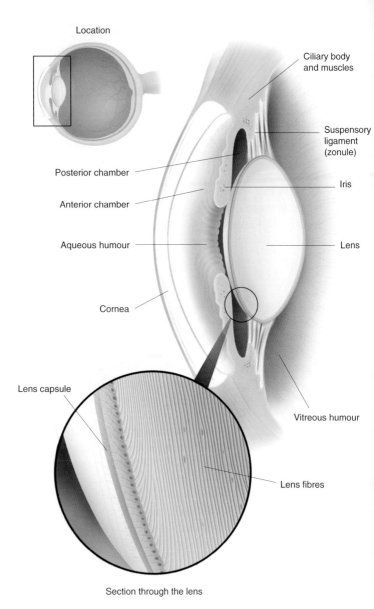

Location

Ciliary body
and muscles

Suspensory
ligament
(zonule)

Posterior chamber

Iris

Anterior chamber

Aqueous humour

Lens

Cornea

Lens capsule

Vitreous humour

Lens fibres

Section through the lens

This illustration shows the detail of the front section of the eye.

with nuclear sclerotic cataracts not to notice the reduction in their visual function until late. The loss of colour appreciation can result in the false assumption that home furnishings are dull in colour or dirty. These are sometimes replaced by more strident colours in order to compensate. After removal of nuclear sclerotic cataracts patients often remark on the brilliance of colours as part of the restoration of their vision.

Cortical cataracts

Cortical cataracts consist of whitish spoke-like opaque patches in the outer part of the lens. They may not

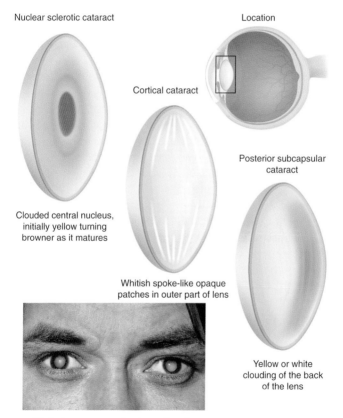

Nuclear sclerotic cataract

Clouded central nucleus, initially yellow turning browner as it matures

Location

Cortical cataract

Whitish spoke-like opaque patches in outer part of lens

Posterior subcapsular cataract

Yellow or white clouding of the back of the lens

Typical appearance of mature cataracts

There are many different forms of cataract, but there are three types that commonly occur as part of the ageing process.

interfere with the central vision for many years, although they can cause dazzle in bright light.

Posterior subcapsular cataracts

Posterior subcapsular cataracts may be associated with ageing, but are also linked with other conditions such as diabetes mellitus and long-term steroid use. This type of cataract mainly affects the outer layer at the back of the lens, may be yellow or white, and can lead to an early deterioration in the vision. Sometimes the vision can be significantly reduced in only a few months.

SYMPTOMS OF CATARACTS

Cataracts are usually found in both eyes, but they are often not at the same stage of development (asymmetrically advanced), so that the vision in one of the eyes may be worse than that of the other. The severity of cataracts varies greatly. Some people may not be aware that a cataract is developing because it can develop at the edge of the lens and initially not cause any symptoms.

People who have small cataracts can often see well enough around the cloudy areas to manage normally. Other people, however, find that they are unable to read, drive or live independently because of the resulting loss of vision. A cataract may cause one or a combination of the following symptoms.

Mistiness or blurring of vision

This usually comes on gradually, although a posterior subcapsular cataract can cause deterioration in your vision over a few weeks. The mistiness is usually spread throughout your field of vision and affects both distance and reading vision. Both of your eyes can be affected, although one is usually worse than the other.

Dazzle, especially in bright sunshine or from car headlights at night

This can be quite disabling but is helped by wearing dark glasses. However, dark glasses will also reduce the amount of light getting into your eye, therefore making the overall level of vision slightly worse.

Reduced colour vision (especially with nuclear sclerotic cataracts)

As cataracts mature and become more yellow or brown, they tend to cut out light, particularly at the blue end of the spectrum, making colours appear dull. After cataract surgery, people are often amazed to find how bright colours can be – for example, in the garden or on home furnishings.

Ghosting of images or double vision

This is most commonly found in people with cortical cataracts. It

As cataracts mature and become more yellow or brown, they tend to cut out light, particularly at the blue end of the spectrum.

usually occurs with each eye separately and therefore is present even with one eye closed. It is often only a minor irritant and does not significantly affect most people with cataracts. Ghosting of the images consists of appreciation of a vague second image of an object which overlaps the main image. This contrasts with frank double vision where two strong images of an object are seen separately.

A shadow in part of your vision

This symptom is occasionally experienced by people with cataracts (particularly of the posterior subcapsular variety). It can also be caused by retinal disease but a visit to the optician/ optometrist should detect the cause.

MAKING A DIAGNOSIS

If your vision is blurred or you have any of the symptoms described above it is advisable to seek help early on in order to establish a definite diagnosis. These symptoms can occasionally be caused by other eye conditions. Initially, make an appointment to see your own

optometrist or doctor. He or she will be able to give you advice regarding the cause of your symptoms and can, if necessary, refer you to an eye specialist (an ophthalmic surgeon) at your local hospital for a more comprehensive eye examination.

A hospital eye specialist will diagnose the kind of cataract you have. You will have a sight test and a full eye examination using a specialist slit-lamp microscope (see page 38). This examination would involve dilating your pupils with drops and this will make your vision blurred for 8 to 10 hours afterwards and it is unwise to drive for this period.

WHEN DO CATARACTS NEED TREATMENT?

Many people with mild cataracts carry on without difficulty. These people do not require any treatment until their vision is affected so that it interferes with their everyday life in some way. Cataracts no longer have to become very dense before surgery can be carried out. In fact, a dense cataract can be more difficult to operate on with the newer small-incision surgery than less-advanced cases.

In many eye units in Britain, there is still a significant waiting list for cataract surgery. Therefore, an early diagnosis can be helpful in preventing a severe loss of vision before cataract surgery can be carried out. If cataracts are left untreated for many years, they may eventually become mature, with the entire lens becoming milky white. Cataracts rarely develop to this maturity in the Western World, although they still commonly occur in developing countries where cataract surgery is not so readily available.

It is especially important to seek early advice if you are suffering from other disabilities, such as hearing loss or poor mobility, because a combination of these with reduced vision can increase the risk of accidents and other problems.

Cataract surgery in developed countries such as Britain is now a relatively safe procedure and is successful in the great majority of cases. However, if other eye diseases (such as macular degeneration) also affect your vision, cataract surgery may not necessarily restore your vision completely. Cataract surgery is discussed in more detail in the next chapter.

DRIVING AND CATARACTS

Driving is often affected early on by cataracts, both as a result of misting of the vision and by dazzle from car headlights or street lighting. The visual acuity only has to be reduced from normal by about 20 per cent to be below the legal limits required in the UK for driving a private motor vehicle. Your optometrist can advise you about this.

KEY POINTS

✓ If you have a cataract, the lens of your eye is cloudy rather than clear

✓ Cataracts have many causes, but most are the result of ageing

✓ Cataracts can cause blurred vision, dazzle, reduced colour vision, double vision and shadows in your vision

✓ Cataract surgery is usually very successful and is a relatively safe procedure

Cataract surgery

If you have a cataract, you may need surgery to improve the vision in your affected eye. This involves removing the lens containing the cataract from your eye and usually replacing it with an artificial lens (called an intraocular lens implant).

TYPES OF SURGERY

Many people think that cataract surgery is carried out with a laser, but this is not actually the case. There are three well-recognised forms of cataract surgery carried out in the world today: phacoemulsification, extracapsular cataract surgery and intracapsular cataract surgery. Most units in Britain have, since the 1990s, taken up the technique of phacoemulsification, as it only uses a small incision and the vision recovers quickly after surgery.

Phacoemulsification

This is the most modern form of cataract surgery and is the operation of choice in most developed countries. The surgical incision used is very small – between 2.6 and 6 millimetres (mm) long. A small incision has many advantages as the surgical wound heals quickly and visual rehabilitation is complete within three to four weeks. Often no stitches (sutures) are required.

Another significant advantage of this type of surgery is the fact that the wound causes little or no post-operative astigmatism (see the chapter on Common sight problems, page 17). Phacoemulsification enables the surgeon to have more control over the pressure within the eye during the operation, preventing collapse of the eye, and reduces the risk of operative complications. Phacoemulsification is suitable for most cataracts, although mature and hard cataractous lenses can be more difficult to remove using this technique.

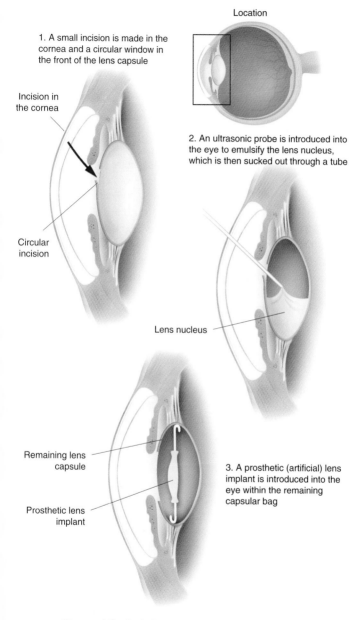

Location

1. A small incision is made in the cornea and a circular window in the front of the lens capsule

Incision in the cornea

Circular incision

2. An ultrasonic probe is introduced into the eye to emulsify the lens nucleus, which is then sucked out through a tube

Lens nucleus

Remaining lens capsule

Prosthetic lens implant

3. A prosthetic (artificial) lens implant is introduced into the eye within the remaining capsular bag

Phacoemulsification is the most modern form of cataract surgery.

At the beginning of the operation, the ophthalmic surgeon makes a small incision in the cornea. Through this, he or she is able to insert small instruments, initially creating a circular window in the front part of the lens capsule. An ultrasonic probe is then introduced into the eye to divide and emulsify (soften and liquefy) the cataractous nucleus of the lens; this can then be sucked out through a small tube. The outer cortical lens matter is removed and, in most cases, a prosthetic (artificial) lens implant is introduced into the eye and placed within the remaining capsular bag thus ensuring that the implant is fixed in the lens' natural position in the eye.

The first lens implant in the world was inserted at St Thomas' Hospital in London in 1949 by a British Ophthalmic Surgeon called Sir Harold Ridley.

There are many types of prosthetic lens and, until recently, lenses made of Perspex were the most common variety. These days, many surgeons prefer to use acrylic or silicone lens implants. This is because these implants can be folded, making it easier to insert them into the eye through the small surgical incision. The implant is then unfolded inside the eye to sit within the capsule bag supported by the curved arms of the lens implant which are known as 'haptics'.

After cataract surgery by phacoemulsification, normal vision has substantially returned within a week, although it usually takes three to four weeks before full rehabilitation occurs and before new spectacles can be prescribed (if they are necessary).

Extracapsular cataract surgery

This form of cataract surgery has been used widely throughout the world since the 1960s and is still practised in many countries. It is still occasionally used in developed countries when the cataractous lens is deemed too difficult to remove by phacoemulsification, for example if the lens is particularly hard in texture. It is an effective form of cataract surgery but involves a larger surgical incision than phacoemulsification. The wound is between 10 and 15 mm in length and requires five or six stitches to close it after the removal of the lens. Surgically induced astigmatism can be a problem, however, requiring removal of the stitches and/or a change of spectacles. Therefore, visual rehabilitation is slower than that achieved with phacoemulsification and may take three months. However, extracapsular cataract surgery is suitable for all kinds of cataractous lenses, even those that are mature or hard in texture.

During extracapsular surgery, a

window is cut in the front surface of the capsule of the lens; through this, the centrally situated nucleus is removed in one piece from the eye and then the surrounding cortical material is vacuumed out using a special suction instrument. In most cases, a prosthetic lens implant is then inserted into the resulting space in the capsular bag. The capsular bag holds the lens implant in the position within the eye normally occupied by the natural lens.

Intracapsular cataract surgery
This operation is now seldom carried out in developed countries, but it may still be necessary in certain circumstances, for instance

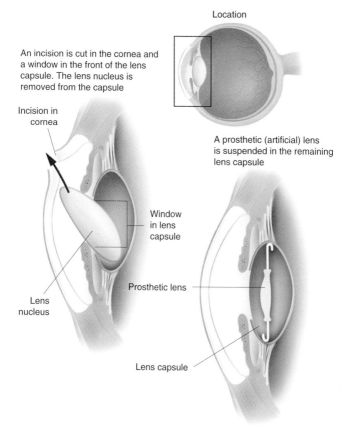

Location

An incision is cut in the cornea and a window in the front of the lens capsule. The lens nucleus is removed from the capsule

Incision in cornea

A prosthetic (artificial) lens is suspended in the remaining lens capsule

Window in lens capsule

Prosthetic lens

Lens nucleus

Lens capsule

Extracapsular cataract surgery is still used when the cataractous lens is deemed too difficult to remove by phacoemulsification.

when the supporting zonules of the lens are too weak. Intracapsular surgery involves the removal of the entire lens, including the outer capsule, which is left in place in phacoemulsification and extra-capsular cataract surgery. Great care is taken to ensure that the front face of the vitreous humour (which lies behind the lens) remains intact so that the vitreous and aqueous humour do not mix as this can lead to complications such as retinal tears and detachments. Lens implantation is still possible but the implant has to be placed in front of the iris and spans the pupil. If a lens is not implanted the vision can be corrected by spectacles but these are very thick and powerful and do

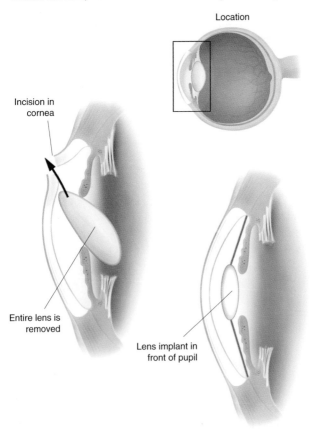

Location

Incision in cornea

Entire lens is removed

Lens implant in front of pupil

Intracapsular cataract surgery involves the removal of the entire lens.

not give a perfect restoration of visual function. In a similar fashion to extracapsular surgery, a relatively large incision is needed together with five or more stitches. Intracapsular surgery is still carried out in many developing countries because the operation is quick and simple, allowing many people to be operated on by a single surgeon in one day. However, the results of intracapsular cataract surgery are not as good as the other two methods described above and it has therefore fallen out of favour in most developed countries.

BENEFITS AND RISKS OF CATARACT SURGERY

As with all forms of surgery, it is important to ensure that the benefits of surgery outweigh the potential risks. If the cataract interferes with your sight so much that the quality of your vision is significantly reduced, then the benefits of cataract surgery can be very great. The risks of surgery, particularly phacoemulsification and extracapsular cataract surgery, are small and about 95 per cent of patients have trouble-free surgery and a successful visual outcome. For the remaining five per cent, complications may occur, but these are frequently minor in nature and usually settle in the first few weeks after surgery. It is advisable to consult your ophthalmic surgeon to discuss the pros and cons of surgery so that a balanced decision can be reached.

ASSESSMENT BEFORE THE OPERATION

Having been referred to an ophthalmic surgeon and diagnosed as having a cataract, your surgeon will carry out a comprehensive examination of your eyes including dilation of your pupils to allow the cataract to be properly assessed and the retina to be looked at to ensure that there are no retinal problems which might be contributing to the reduction in your vision. If your pupils do have to be dilated this will blur your vision and preclude driving for 8 to 10 hours. Some people with cataracts also have coexisting macular disease (see the chapter on page 69), which may prevent the return of perfect vision even after the cataract has been removed. Nevertheless, in many cases, the removal of the cataract can improve the vision substantially and is still worthwhile. Your eye surgeon will be able to advise you about this.

Once surgery has been decided on, the surgeon will need to carry out a number of tests. These will enable him or her to decide what power of intraocular lens should be implanted into your eye. These tests are straightforward and painless, and involve measuring the curvature of the front surface of your cornea and also the length of your eye (using a painless ultrasonic or infrared measure). This process is called 'biometry'.

The power of the intraocular lens implant selected is the one that is most appropriate to your current spectacle prescription and desired postoperative refraction (power of the glasses). By implanting an artificial lens, the surgeon can significantly reduce, or even eliminate, long-sightedness or short-sightedness in people who have previously had to wear strong spectacles. The surgeon will discuss with you the postoperative refraction you wish to have and will aim to achieve this by selecting an appropriate lens implant power. The choice of the postoperative refraction aimed for is dictated by the power of the spectacle lens in the other eye because it is important not to create an imbalance between the two eyes by having one spectacle lens that is very powerful and the other with little power. This is called 'anisometropia'. In addition some people who have been short-

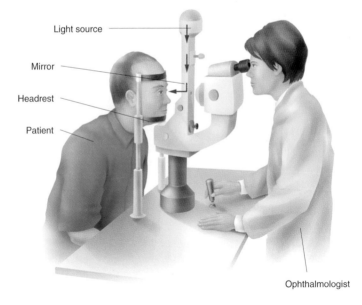

Light source

Mirror

Headrest

Patient

Ophthalmologist

A slit lamp produces a narrow beam of intense light that allows examination of the structures of the eye. The pupils must be fully dilated with eyedrops if the retina is to be thoroughly examined.

sighted (myopic) all their lives prefer to stay short-sighted, although many like to take the opportunity to eliminate or reduce this. If the refraction is set to be neutral for distance, then spectacles will still be required for reading.

As we get older the natural lens inside the eye becomes less malleable and will therefore not change shape to accommodate for reading. This is why we need reading glasses in middle age and later. Therefore replacing the natural lens with a lens implant that has a fixed focus does not create problems for the older recipient. There have been a number of trials of bifocal intraocular lenses but these have not, as yet, proved popular because of the difficulty of achieving good vision for both distance and near vision.

Biometry is usually carried out a day or two before surgery. Your consultant will also check for any possible sources of infection from your eyelids (blepharitis), conjunctiva (conjunctivitis) or elsewhere such as urinary infections or leg ulcers. These sources of infection would need to be treated with antibiotics before surgery in order to reduce the risk of infectious contamination during the operation. The consultant will also carry out a general assessment of the eye and will check the state of the retina.

The anaesthetist will assess your

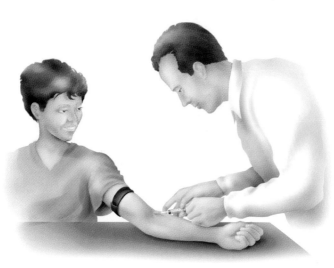

It may be necessary for you to have blood taken for tests.

general health and appropriateness for a local or general anaesthetic. Many parts of the preoperative assessment may also be carried out by a suitably trained nurse. It may be necessary for you to have blood taken for tests and to have an electrocardiogram (ECG), especially if a general anaesthetic is being considered. If you are allergic to any medications, drops or sticking plaster, it is important to notify your pre-assessment nurse, surgeon and anaesthetist of this.

DAY-CASE OR INPATIENT SURGERY?

Cataract surgery is usually straightforward and should not cause you any constitutional upset. It can be carried out on a day-case basis or as an inpatient (overnight stay). With day-case surgery, you come in on the day of the surgery a few hours before the operation and can go home the same day after having been seen by the surgeon on his or her postoperative ward round. Your eye usually requires a postoperative

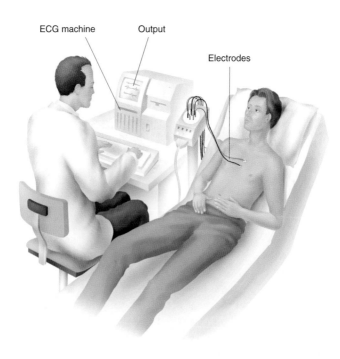

ECG machine   Output

Electrodes

Before general anaesthesia, an electrocardiogram (ECG) is often required. An ECG is used to record the electrical activity of the heart.

QUESTIONS TO ASK YOUR CONSULTANT

1. How straightforward is this procedure?
2. Do I have any other eye diseases that could affect the outcome of the operation?
3. Do I have any health problems that could complicate matters?
4. Will you be inserting a lens implant and, if so, which type?
5. Will I be able to have day-case surgery?
6. Will I have a local or general anaesthetic?
7. What are my chances of having poorer vision after the operation or losing the sight in the eye?
8. I am taking regular medications. On the day of surgery when should I take them?
9. Can I eat or drink before surgery. If not, when do I have to stop?
10. How long will the healing process take?
11. Will I have to wear glasses or contact lenses afterwards? If so, when?
12. Are there any activities I should avoid afterwards?

check-up the next day at the hospital; this is carried out by your surgeon or a trained nurse and in some centres is achieved by phoning you at home to ask how you are getting on. If day-case surgery is being considered, it is important that you are well with no serious conditions, such as angina or severe chest disease, and that you have home support available for the night after the operation, together with private transport to and from the hospital. Although most day-case cataract surgery is carried out under a local anaesthetic, having a general anaesthetic does not preclude a day-case stay.

If you have no home support, are infirm or have a significant medical condition, inpatient surgery will probably be more appropriate. You may come in on the day before your operation or sometimes on the day itself and usually stay for one night afterwards. The decision about whether cataract surgery should be carried out as a day case or with an overnight stay will be made with your eye surgeon and anaesthetist.

THE ANAESTHETIC

Cataract surgery can be carried out under either a local anaesthetic or a general anaesthetic. Most patients have a local anaesthetic, but the decision depends on your preference and the advice of your eye surgeon and anaesthetist.

Local anaesthetic

If you have a local anaesthetic, it is given by an injection through either your conjunctiva or the skin beneath the eye so that the anaesthetic bathes the area around the eye and prevents it from feeling anything or moving during the operation. One or two injections may be necessary. Under some circumstances, the local anaesthetic may also prevent your eye seeing anything during surgery. Even if this is not the case, most patients are aware of only vague shadows in their field of view during the operation. The local anaesthetic injection takes three to five hours to wear off after the operation. You may be asked not to eat for four to five hours before the operation and not to drink for two hours, but it is important to find out from your anaesthetist and surgeon the particular protocol that they adopt. Some surgeons carry out cataract surgery using topical anaesthesia. This involves using anaesthetic drops on your eye, which prevent feeling but allow the eye to move normally. This is a simple approach which avoids an injection and is preferred by some people. Additional anaesthesia can be administered during the operation if necessary. Premedications (such as sedatives or tranquillisers) are not usually necessary and may not be desirable as they may cause you to fall asleep and wake with a start during surgery.

General anaesthetic

If you have a general anaesthetic, you may be given premedication an hour or so before surgery and you will be unconscious throughout the operation. General anaesthesia for cataract surgery does not have to be particularly deep, and the post-operative recovery period is usually quick, with little nausea or after-effects.

If you are taking medicines for heart disease or high blood pressure, it is important that you take them on the day of your operation. Patients having a general anaesthetic will be asked to have nothing to eat or drink for five or more hours before the operation.

THE OPERATION

During the hour before surgery, one of the nurses on the ward will administer drops to the eye in order to dilate (widen) the pupil. This is to enable the surgeon to remove the cataractous lens through the dilated pupil. If you are having your operation under a local anaesthetic, it is important to wear your hearing aid (if you have one) and you do not need to remove any false teeth.

Modern cataract surgery usually takes half an hour or less. During the operation, you will be lying flat on the operating table and the position of the table can be altered to make you more comfortable. It is important that you remain calm and still during the procedure. A paper or cloth drape is placed over your head, face and chest. This is held away from your nose and mouth, and fresh air and oxygen are fed in under the drapes so that you can breathe comfortably.

If you are having a local anaesthetic, a nurse will hold your hand throughout the operation. This is a natural source of comfort, but also acts as a form of communication between you and your surgeon. If you wish to speak or move, then squeezing the nurse's hand twice will enable the nurse to tell your surgeon to pause and find out what you wish to say.

The eyelids of the eye being operated upon are held open by a prop during the operation; you therefore do not need to be concerned about blinking and can close the other eye.

To remove the cataractous lens, the surgeon will use an operating microscope which incorporates a bright light that shines onto your eye but does not usually cause any discomfort. At the end of the operation, the surgeon will apply antibiotics and/or sterilising drops to your eye, and a pad or shield will be placed over the operated eye and stuck to the face with adhesive tape.

POSTOPERATIVE RECOVERY AND TREATMENT

Immediately after the operation, you will be taken to the recovery bay before going back to the ward. If a local anaesthetic was used, you may be able simply to go straight back to the ward in a wheelchair or sit in an armchair in the recovery area. After recovery, you can have a drink and something to eat and, if you are being treated as a day case, you can go home.

Sometimes, you will be asked to take tablets to prevent a pressure rise in your eye during the immediate postoperative period. The eye shield or pad will remain in place until your eye has been checked by the surgeon or nurse the next day. Your level of vision is usually measured on the first postoperative day, and the vision may be bright but not necessarily very sharp at this stage. The vision usually recovers quickly during the first few days after surgery. Sometimes patients do not have to come back to the hospital the day after surgery. Instead, he or she is telephoned by a specialist nurse to ensure that the eye is settling satisfactorily and to give advice.

After the surgery there may be some discomfort in the eye but there is not normally any significant pain. Simple analgesic tablets may be taken if the eye is uncomfortable. If the eye has significant pain then you should bring this to the attention of the nursing staff on the ward or telephone the hospital if you are already at home. If you have had a local anaesthetic you may experience some double vision as the anaesthetic wears off but this usually resolves within six to eight hours of the operation. The eye may be light sensitive for a few days after the operation and it is wise to have a pair of dark glasses to hand in case this happens. The nurse who has been looking after you on the ward will advise you about the care of your eye after your operation. Some advice on various points is set out below.

Drops

Most patients will be given antibiotic and anti-inflammatory drops to put in the eye for a few weeks after the operation. These drops reduce eye inflammation and prevent infection. Detailed instructions will be given to you before discharge. Most people are able to apply these drops themselves, but if you find it difficult a relative or district nurse can help.

Outpatient appointment

You will usually be seen as an outpatient once or twice after the operation, commonly one week after surgery and again three to four weeks later.

If your eye aches or your vision deteriorates, this may be a sign of a potential problem with your eye and you should quickly contact the eye ward or your surgeon to ask for advice.

Work, housework and cooking

You should avoid heavy lifting and straining for about four weeks after surgery, but otherwise you can carry on as normal. Most people can return to their jobs after two weeks.

Bending

You may bend normally but take care not to knock your eye.

Driving

It is best to avoid driving, at least until after your first outpatient visit, when you can ask the surgeon if your vision is good enough.

At night

Most surgeons will ask you to wear a protective eye shield over the operated eye for the first week after surgery.

Bathing

For the first week, avoid getting the eye wet and avoid rubbing, touching or pressing on the eye. You may wash your hair or go to the hairdresser but should wear your protective eye shield for this.

Spectacles

Immediately after your operation, your vision may be blurred. You can wear your present spectacles (or dark glasses) if they help, but you will probably need a change of spectacles about three to four weeks after surgery. You will be asked to go to your optometrist for these.

Stitches

Occasionally you require stitches for your eye wound after surgery. These are commonly made of nylon and are usually inert (non-reactive). They are often removed in the first few months after the operation.

The removal of the stitches is very straightforward and is carried out as an outpatient procedure using anaesthetic drops. If the stitches are not removed, sometimes, months or years after the operation, the stitches can break causing a foreign body sensation in the eye. If this happens, the broken stitch or stitches can be removed by an eye surgeon using an examining microscope – this is also an outpatient procedure carried out under local anaesthetic drops.

POSSIBLE COMPLICATIONS

Complications during and after cataract surgery are rare, and 95 per cent of patients have trouble-free operations. In a small number of cases (usually one per cent or less), the membrane within the eye (the posterior capsule) may break during the operation, enabling the vitreous humour (the jelly within the back part of the eye) to come forward. Usually it is straightforward to remove the vitreous humour surgically at the time of the cataract operation so that a lens implant can be successfully inserted into the eye and the vision restored. If the vitreous humour is removed it is replaced by fluid.

Occasionally there is some bleeding beneath the surface of your eye (subconjunctival haemorrhage) and, although this looks dramatic, it usually clears up without difficulty within a week or two and does not affect the outcome of the operation.

In the first few days after the operation, the eye can become inflamed (called uveitis or iritis). This generally clears up when treated with anti-inflammatory drops.

Another possible complication is the onset of water logging at the central part of the retina (macular oedema). This consists of an accumulation of fluid within the layers of the retina at the macula and is more common if the posterior capsule has ruptured during the operation. This can affect your detailed vision but once again frequently clears up after a few weeks.

A rare but serious complication can occur if the inside of the operated eye becomes infected (endophthalmitis). This occurs in between one in 400 and one in 1,000 patients. It usually occurs within a few days of the operation and is characterised by the onset of severe aching in, and/or around, the eye and is associated with blurring of the vision. If these symptoms do occur, it is important to contact your eye surgeon or the eye ward immediately to ask for advice. If caught early enough, intensive treatment with antibiotics can clear up the infection and give a good visual outcome.

In some cases the membrane that lies behind the lens implant (the posterior capsule) may become cloudy (opaque) after the operation.

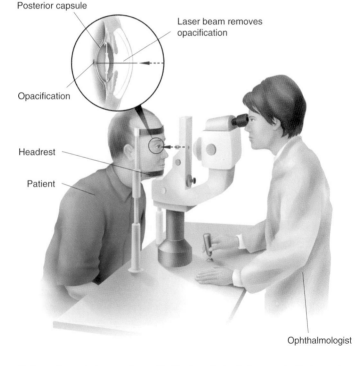

Posterior capsule

Laser beam removes opacification

Opacification

Headrest

Patient

Ophthalmologist

Postoperative posterior capsule opacification is easily treated as an outpatient procedure using a laser and examination microscope.

If this happens, it generally takes at least six months to appear. The likelihood of this happening depends on a number of factors, including your age and the type of lens implant used. It occurs more commonly in young people and is less common with acrylic lenses (approximately 2.5 per cent of cases) but more common with Perspex lenses (approximately 35 per cent of cases). There are many different kinds of implants used and if you are concerned about this point you should discuss the issue with your eye surgeon. Opacification of the posterior capsule results in a misting of the vision, similar to that occurring with the original cataract. Fortunately it is easily treated as an outpatient procedure using a laser mounted on an examination microscope. It is carried out using local anaesthetic drops and a contact lens and takes about 10 minutes.

After the laser treatment, the vision is restored and further clouding of the posterior capsule does not usually occur. The procedure is straightforward and is easily tolerated even by elderly or infirm people. Complications are rare, although there is a small increase in the risk of developing a retinal tear, detachment or cystoid macular oedema (mentioned above).

I have described most of the complications that can occur with cataract surgery. Reading about these complications could unnerve you, so remember that for the vast majority of people cataract surgery is straightforward and leads to an excellent visual result.

SPECTACLES AND REFRACTION

If the cataract has been removed using the phacoemulsification technique, the eye will be sufficiently well healed three to six weeks after surgery to enable you to have a change of spectacles if necessary. If extracapsular surgery has been carried out, however, you must wait for two to three months after the surgery before you consider new spectacles. This is because the surgical wound in extracapsular surgery is much larger and takes longer to heal. The prosthetic lens implant cannot change its power in the way that a natural lens can (although in elderly people this ability is much reduced). You therefore usually require spectacles for reading and for fine tuning of the distance vision. Varifocal lenses or bifocal lenses (described above) may be appropriate and this should be discussed with your optometrist.

During your preoperative assessment and biometry (see above), your eye surgeon will have selected the power of the lens implant to suit your needs. This may mean that the spectacles you require postoperatively will be much less powerful than those used before surgery or they may not be necessary at all for distance vision.

Your surgeon will either refract your eye (assess any optical errors) himself or give you a note to take to your optometrist for refraction and the supply of spectacles. There may be some changes in the prescription you need over the first few months after surgery and it is wise to visit your optometrist for a further check-up about six months after the operation.

KEY POINTS

✓ Cataract surgery involves removing the cloudy lens and replacing it with an implant

✓ Phacoemulsification is the most common type of cataract surgery. It uses a very small incision and most patients recover their vision very quickly

✓ Surgery can be a day-case or inpatient procedure and may be performed under a local or general anaesthetic

✓ Most patients return to their normal routine quickly, and complications are rare

Glaucoma

Glaucoma is a leading cause of blindness in the UK. It tends to affect people over 40 years old and, in most cases, there are no warning symptoms until the late stages. Blindness can be prevented if the condition is diagnosed and treated early on. For this reason, it is essential that you have regular eye examinations.

If you have been diagnosed with glaucoma, ask your eye specialist to explain the condition and treatment to you and to outline the possible effects of the condition in the future.

WHAT IS GLAUCOMA?

The term 'glaucoma' is used to describe a group of eye conditions characterised by damage to the optic nerve within the eye, resulting in a loss of visual field. This process is generally very gradual and is usually associated with a higher than normal pressure within the eye (intraocular pressure or IOP). If the pressure is too high, the optic nerve can be damaged.

There are two main types of glaucoma: open-angle glaucoma and angle-closure glaucoma. Open-angle glaucoma comes on gradually (a chronic condition) and there are no warning symptoms until there has been considerable damage to the optic nerve and associated loss of the visual field. Angle-closure glaucoma is much more sudden in onset (an acute condition) and produces severe symptoms.

To understand the difference between these two forms, it is necessary to know about the production and drainage of fluid in the front chamber of the eye. This fluid (aqueous humour) is continuously produced within the eye by the ciliary body, which lies in the midpoint of the eye close to the lens (see page 52). The fluid passes forwards through the pupil and drains away through tiny drainage channels into the bloodstream.

One source of drainage is called the trabecular meshwork, which is responsible for most of the fluid outflow and the other is the uveoscleral pathway. The trabecular meshwork is found in the angle where the iris meets the cornea (an area called the drainage angle). Normally, the amount of fluid produced is the same as the amount of fluid draining out. However, if the fluid cannot escape, or too much is produced, the eye pressure will rise.

TYPES OF GLAUCOMA

Open-angle glaucoma

In this form, the drainage angle is open but does not allow enough fluid to drain away from within your eye, either because the drainage angle is partially blocked or because the eye produces too much aqueous humour. The fluid therefore builds up and causes a rise in the pressure within the eye. This pressure rise is usually slow and painless.

Angle-closure (closed-angle) glaucoma

In this form, the drainage angle becomes closed by the iris and the fluid is unable to drain away from the eye. This usually happens quite quickly and the pressure rise is much greater than that of open-

angle glaucoma. It is usually accompanied by significant symptoms such as marked aching in the eye and blurring. These symptoms are described in more detail below. Angle-closure glaucoma is a medical emergency and must be treated immediately.

Ocular hypertension

Some people have an open drainage angle and a moderate rise in intraocular pressure but no other signs of open-angle glaucoma such as optic nerve damage or visual field loss. The upper limit of normal pressure is defined as 21 millimetres of mercury (mmHg). In some people, the pressure may be higher than this and still be normal for them, whereas in others, pressures of over 21 mmHg may be an early sign of glaucoma. If someone has high intraocular pressure without having other signs of glaucoma, they are classed as having 'ocular hypertension'. These people do not require eye treatment unless they show the other signs of developing glaucoma (peripheral field loss and/or optic disc cupping) or have predisposing factors such as a positive family history of glaucoma. They are monitored regularly to see if further signs develop.

Other forms of glaucoma

There are many different kinds of

glaucoma other than those described above, but they are rare and do not merit detailed consideration here. So-called secondary glaucoma can occur as a result of other conditions within the eye such as inflammation (uveitis or iritis). Developmental glaucoma in babies is caused by a malformation in the eye of the fetus in the uterus and is very rare in the UK.

OPEN-ANGLE GLAUCOMA

Causes
The specific cause of chronic open-angle glaucoma ('chronic' means continuing for a long time) is unknown. However, it seems to be a combination of higher than normal pressure within the eye and a less effective blood supply to your optic nerve. The intraocular pressure rise is thought to result from a reduced ability of the drainage angle to drain away the fluid within the eye.

There are a number of factors (described below) that increase the risk of developing open-angle glaucoma. It is not possible to prevent the condition from developing, but early diagnosis and careful treatment can help to prevent or slow its progression. Most optometrists in the UK will routinely test you for possible glaucoma and refer you to the hospital eye service if they are suspicious. It is therefore wise to

visit your optometrist at least every two years for a test. If you have a first-degree relative (mother, father, sister, brother or child) with the condition, you should have an annual check-up and you will not be charged for it.

The main risk factors for chronic open-angle glaucoma include the following.

- **Older age:** Open-angle glaucoma is much more common with increasing age. It is rare below the age of 40 but affects one per cent of the population aged 40 and above, and five per cent of people over the age of 65.

- **Positive family history:** If you have a first-degree relative with the condition, you are at an increased risk of developing it yourself. This risk has not been accurately defined, but is in the region of one in five. Everyone who has a first-degree relative with glaucoma should have their intraocular pressure monitored annually by their optometrist (no charge is made for this examination).

- **Short-sightedness (myopia):** People who are short-sighted are more likely to develop glaucoma than others.

- **Race:** People of African origin have a greater risk of developing

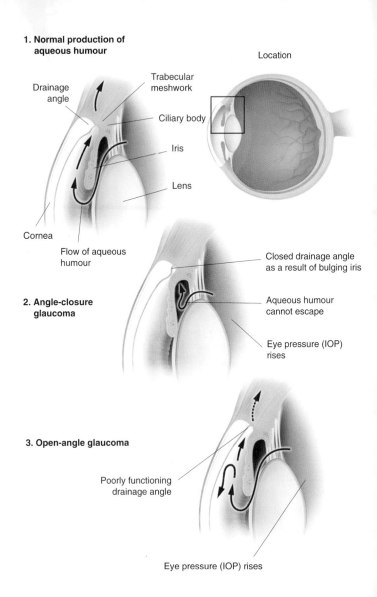

1. Normal production of aqueous humour

Drainage angle

Trabecular meshwork

Ciliary body

Iris

Lens

Cornea

Flow of aqueous humour

Location

2. Angle-closure glaucoma

Closed drainage angle as a result of bulging iris

Aqueous humour cannot escape

Eye pressure (IOP) rises

3. Open-angle glaucoma

Poorly functioning drainage angle

Eye pressure (IOP) rises

Glaucoma is usually associated with a higher than normal pressure within the eye. If the pressure is too high, the optic nerve can be damaged.

chronic open-angle glaucoma. The condition may develop at a younger age than in other people.

Symptoms of chronic open-angle glaucoma

If you have chronic open-angle glaucoma, you may not actually notice any symptoms, unless the condition is very advanced, in which case you may notice some loss in the visual field. The condition is entirely painless and the central vision is generally preserved until the disease is at an advanced stage.

Damage that has already been done to the retinal nerve fibres and optic nerve by the time the glaucoma is diagnosed cannot be reversed. However, with early diagnosis and careful treatment, the damage can usually be restricted and the progression of the disease halted or slowed down. If untreated, chronic open-angle glaucoma can eventually lead to a severe loss of vision or even blindness. Therefore early diagnosis and treatment are vital.

Making a diagnosis

The diagnosis of chronic open-angle glaucoma is based on three main factors:

1. Raised pressure within the eye (usually greater than 21 mmHg).
2. Characteristic loss of visual field, although you may not notice this.
3. Cupping of the optic nerve

within the eye (where the optic nerve head becomes concave as a result of the loss of nerve fibres).

The diagnosis of chronic open-angle glaucoma is commonly made by a hospital eye specialist after referral from an optometrist and/or a GP. The three tests for glaucoma are:

- **Optic nerve head assessment:** The retina and optic nerve are examined by shining a light from a special instrument (ophthalmoscope) into the eye or examining the eye with a special lens in conjunction with a biomicroscope (a slit lamp). Cupping and paleness of the optic nerve head in the eye are characteristic signs of glaucoma.

- **Tonometry:** The intraocular pressure is measured using a special instrument called a tonometer. In hospital eye departments this involves the application of anaesthetic drops and is a quick simple procedure and once again is carried out using the slit-lamp biomicroscope. Many optometrists (opticians) use a different method of measuring the pressure, using a puff of air directed towards the eye.

- **Perimetry:** The visual field is examined to look for any loss in the peripheral vision. This is achieved using a perimeter for which you

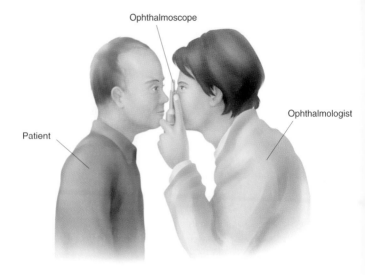

Ophthalmoscope

Ophthalmologist

Patient

An ophthalmoscope is used to examine the retina and optic nerve.

need to sit with your chin on a rest looking straight at a small target. Spots of light of varying intensity are presented in the periphery of the visual field and you are asked to indicate by pressing a buzzer when the spot is seen. The procedure is straightforward and takes approximately five minutes for each eye.

TREATMENT OF CHRONIC OPEN-ANGLE GLAUCOMA

Medication

The treatment for chronic open-angle glaucoma is to reduce the pressure within the eye. This is frequently achieved with eyedrops. There are many different kinds of drops that can be used to lower the intraocular pressure. Generally one type of drop will be tried initially and, if this does not lower the intraocular pressure sufficiently, further drops may be added.

Please note that the proper (or generic) names are used in this text to describe drops and other medications. Most medications are also known by their commercial (or proprietary) names which are different from the proper names. Please ask the chemist if in doubt.

There can be side effects from the drops, although these are not usually serious. However, you should read the instruction leaflet with the drops and tell your specialist if you have asthma or other chest problems or vascular or heart disease, as not all drops will be suitable. Some of the drops are believed to increase the blood supply to the optic nerve within your eye as well as lowering the pressure. The drops used for chronic open-angle glaucoma include the following.

• **Prostaglandins:** These are hormone-like substances that keep your blood vessels dilated (widened) so that more fluid can flow through them. Examples used to treat glaucoma are called latanoprost, travoprost and bimatoprost. They lower the pressure in the eye by increasing the outflow of the aqueous humour from the eye.

Side effects: prostaglandin drops appear to have few significant side effects on the body as a whole, but can cause the eyelashes to darken and lengthen and/or the iris to darken in colour.

• **Beta blockers:** These drops are commonly used for glaucoma. They lower the pressure inside the eye, probably by reducing the production of aqueous fluid. The beta blockers used in eyedrops for glaucoma are called betaxolol, carteolol, levobunolol, metipranolol and timolol.

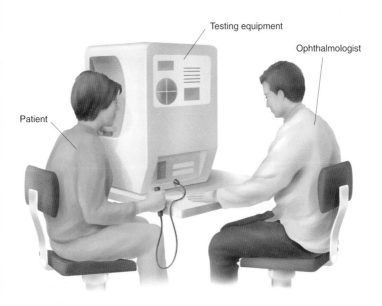

Testing equipment

Ophthalmologist

Patient

Perimetry or visual field testing is used to look for any loss in the peripheral vision, measuring the whole area that the eye can see.

Side effects: beta blockers can precipitate or exacerbate asthma or other forms of chest disease (such as chronic obstructive pulmonary disease) and are contraindicated in people with chest disease. More rarely they can cause a slowing of the pulse and should be used with caution in patients who are using other heart medications (particularly beta-blocker tablets). Furthermore, they are contraindicated in people with peripheral blood vessel disease causing cold hands and feet. They can also sometimes make the eyes feel dry and have been reported to cause sleepiness and lethargy.

- **Miotics:** These drops contract the iris muscles and constrict the pupil. This pulls the iris away from the trabecular meshwork and allows the fluid to drain away more readily. The drugs used are called carbachol and pilocarpine.

Side effects: as miotics affect the pupil and the accommodation of the lens, they can interfere with reading vision and also make distance vision blurred. They can also cause the eye to ache for 20 to 30 minutes after administration. These side effects often fade with continuing use. Miotic drops can make it more difficult to see in dark conditions because of the constriction of the pupil and, over a long period of time, can predispose to the development of cataracts. Miotics are not used very frequently nowadays in the treatment of open-angle glaucoma, although they are one of the treatments of choice in the angle-closure variety (see page 58).

- **Sympathomimetics:** These drugs are believed to act by reducing the production of aqueous humour and by increasing the outflow through the trabecular meshwork. They are called adrenaline (epinephrine), dipivefrine and guanethidine.

Side effects: these drops tend to cause the superficial blood vessels of the eye to dilate, making the eye look red. Over a long period of time they have also been known to cause scarring beneath the conjunctiva.

- **Carbonic anhydrase inhibitors:** These drops reduce the production of aqueous humour by the ciliary body. They are called brinzolamide and dorzolamide. Carbonic anhydrase inhibitors are also available in tablet form (as acetazolamide) and these act by reducing the fluid levels in the body.

Side effects: if used for long periods the tablet form can cause an imbalance in the salts of the body (potassium loss), and blood tests need to be carried two or three times a year to check that this imbalance is not occurring. In addition, carbonic anhydrase inhibitors commonly cause tingling of the extremities (in particular the fingers and toes).

• **Alpha-2 agonists:** These drugs, brimonidine and apraclonidine, reduce the production of the aqueous humour from the ciliary body.

Side effects: in approximately 15 per cent of cases these drops can cause marked allergic reactions in the eyes and cause redness and discomfort. This reaction may not occur until six months after starting the drops.

If the glaucoma cannot be controlled with drops alone, short-term control can be achieved with tablets. The most notable of these is a carbonic anhydrase inhibitor (see above) called acetazolamide, which acts by powerfully reducing the amount of fluid (aqueous humour) produced within your eye, thereby lowering the pressure. However, it has a number of side effects – for example, tingling in the fingers and toes – and can lead to a reduction in your body's potassium level. It is therefore generally used only for short periods unless under the close supervision of the medical ophthalmic specialist or GP.

Surgical treatments
If drugs fail to help your glaucoma, the specialist may suggest either laser treatment or an operation called trabeculectomy to improve the drainage of fluid from the eye. For more details of these procedures, please see Surgery for open-angle glaucoma (page 62).

Monitoring glaucoma
Most people with glaucoma are reviewed by their eye specialist two or three times a year. At each consultation, the intraocular pressure will be measured and the condition of the optic nerve will be checked by the specialist looking inside the eye with the help of a bright light from the biomicroscope and a special lens.

The visual fields will be tested every year (possibly more frequently soon after the diagnosis) and photographs may be taken of the optic nerve head for your medical records.

ANGLE-CLOSURE GLAUCOMA

Causes
Acute angle-closure glaucoma ('acute' means it arises suddenly) is more common in people who are very long-sighted (hypermetropic), and these people may have worn spectacles since childhood. The condition is more common over the age of 40 and affects more women than men.

There are a variety of medicines that can increase the risk of angle-closure glaucoma, especially major tranquillisers used in the treatment of depression and other psychiatric conditions. Your doctor will advise you about the medicines that can predispose to the development of acute angle-closure glaucoma. You should also read the manufacturer's leaflet that accompanies your medicines to see whether they could trigger acute glaucoma.

Symptoms

In marked contrast to the lack of symptoms in early open-angle glaucoma, angle-closure glaucoma usually has many symptoms. Early symptoms may consist of mild aching in the eye, associated with blurred vision and sometimes seeing coloured rainbow effects around lights. These symptoms are more common in dim light or darkness and often resolve after a night's sleep. If you are suffering from these symptoms, a visit to your optometrist may be helpful so that your eye can be examined for any factors that predispose to the development of angle-closure glaucoma.

In a severe attack, the pressure increase in the eye can be great and occur over a few hours. The eye becomes very painful with a marked ache that may extend around the eye to the brow and temple. It usually affects only one eye at a time. The eye becomes red, and the

vision deteriorates and is blurred. The affected person may also experience nausea and vomiting. If these symptoms occur, you need an urgent referral to the hospital eye service. You can get this referral through either your GP or your optometrist.

Making a diagnosis

Although this is a relatively unusual disease, a busy eye unit in the UK will see one or two cases of acute angle-closure glaucoma per week. The diagnosis is readily made on the symptoms described above, together with a markedly raised intraocular pressure measured using tonometry. The diagnosis is established in the hospital eye accident and emergency department, but your optometrist or GP will probably have suspected the diagnosis when they arranged an urgent referral.

Treatment

The high pressure in the eye can be readily treated with drops and medicines, which are initially administered in the eye accident and emergency department. The medicines most commonly used are pilocarpine drops (see page 56) and acetazolamide (often given by injection into a vein). In addition you will be given painkillers and treatment for nausea and vomiting if necessary. The intraocular pressure is usually reduced within a few hours, but most people are admitted to hospital for their treatment and to monitor the pressure after this. Most patients stay in hospital for only a few days. Steroid or other anti-inflammatory drops to reduce the accompanying inflammation in the eye are also usually given.

When the eye pressure is back to normal and the eye is less inflamed, laser treatment is given to prevent future attacks of angle-closure glaucoma. The laser is used to make a small hole in the peripheral part of the iris, to allow the fluid (aqueous humour) to drain away without having to pass through the pupil. This treatment is called a 'peripheral iridotomy'. It is a simple procedure that is often carried out in the outpatient department. It involves giving anaesthetic drops and placing a contact lens on the eye to provide a magnified view of the iris. The laser treatment is delivered using a slit-lamp biomicroscope similar to the one used to examine the eye. The unaffected eye may also be treated

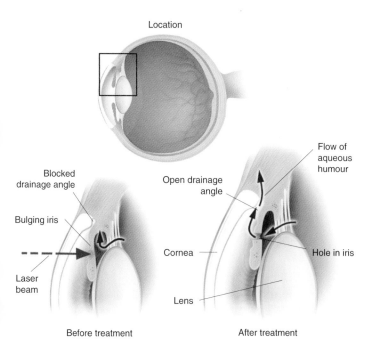

Location

Blocked drainage angle

Bulging iris

Laser beam

Open drainage angle

Flow of aqueous humour

Cornea

Hole in iris

Lens

Before treatment

After treatment

Peripheral iridotomy is used to treat acute glaucoma. A laser is used to make a small hole in the peripheral part of the iris to allow the aqueous humour to drain through.

with a laser to prevent the development of an acute attack in this eye.

If diagnosed and treated early, acute angle-closure glaucoma does not lead to any significant damage to the vision, optic nerve or visual fields. The laser treatment described above usually prevents further attacks. Further substantive treatment is needed only in a minority of patients who suffer from recurrent pressure rises. This often involves a surgical procedure similar to that carried out in chronic open-angle glaucoma (a trabeculectomy, see page 62).

DRIVING AND GLAUCOMA

To reach the legal requirements to drive in the UK, your visual fields must be substantially normal. If your visual field has been damaged by glaucoma of any kind, you may fall below the required limits and your licence and insurance will not be valid. It is necessary for anyone who drives and has glaucoma to inform the Driver and Vehicle Licensing Agency (DVLA) at Swansea. Your eye consultant or optometrist will then be asked to assess your visual function for driving and advise you accordingly.

KEY POINTS

✓ Glaucoma involves damage to your optic nerve and is usually associated with raised pressure within your eye

✓ Open-angle (chronic) glaucoma progresses slowly with few symptoms and is most common with advancing age and in people with a family history of the condition

✓ Open-angle glaucoma can be treated with eyedrops, tablets or, if these fail to work, surgery

✓ Angle-closure (acute) glaucoma is sudden in onset and painful; it is treated as a medical emergency

✓ Angle-closure glaucoma is treated with eyedrops and intravenous medicines, and later laser therapy to prevent future attacks

Surgery for open-angle glaucoma

If you have chronic open-angle glaucoma, you may need to have surgery if your intraocular pressure is not being controlled well enough by drops or other medicines.

TYPES OF SURGERY

The most common operation carried out in developed countries is called a trabeculectomy, although laser treatment may also be used. Your eye specialist will discuss with you which method of treatment is the best in your particular case. Surgery can be carried out as a day-case or an overnight procedure (as an inpatient) and, in a similar way to cataract surgery, it is often performed under a local anaesthetic.

Trabeculectomy

Trabeculectomy results in the formation of a water blister (bleb) on the surface of the eye beneath the eyelid. It is formed by drawing back a flap of conjunctiva and then creating a trapdoor flap within the white scleral coat of the eye. This allows the fluid to drain out of the eye in a controlled fashion. Stitches are usually required but these biodegrade and disappear after a few weeks. The operation is usually very successful in controlling the pressure in the eye for a considerable period of time, sometimes many years.

Trabeculectomy is suitable for most varieties of glaucoma but it is used only after medical treatment in the form of drops and medicines has failed to control the intraocular pressure. The formation of the trabeculectomy bleb is combined with fashioning of a hole in the peripheral part of the iris (a peripheral iridectomy), which allows the aqueous fluid to drain from the ciliary body to the front part of the inside of the eye without having to pass through the pupil.

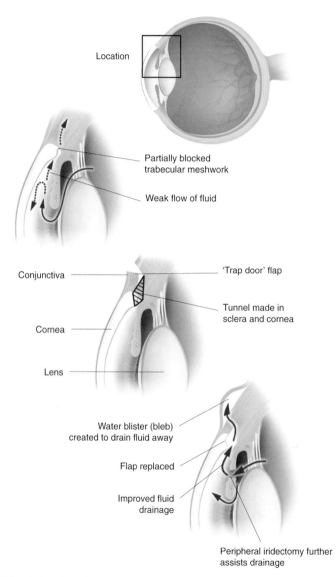

Location

Partially blocked
trabecular meshwork

Weak flow of fluid

Conjunctiva

'Trap door' flap

Tunnel made in
sclera and cornea

Cornea

Lens

Water blister (bleb)
created to drain fluid away

Flap replaced

Improved fluid
drainage

Peripheral iridectomy further
assists drainage

Trabeculectomy is used to treat open-angle glaucoma. A trapdoor flap is created in the
white scleral coat of the eye. This allows the fluid produced in the eye to drain away in
a controlled fashion.

Laser treatment

There are various forms of laser treatment available for open-angle glaucoma. Until recently one prevalent form of laser treatment was laser trabeculoplasty (LTP). This involves using an argon gas laser administered under local anaesthetic drops and using a contact lens to view the drainage angle of the eye (the trabecular meshwork). The laser is applied to the trabecular meshwork and is said to work by opening up the pores of the meshwork, thereby allowing the aqueous fluid to drain more readily from the eye. This procedure is less popular now.

Another form of laser treatment (a diode laser) is more commonly used these days, but is reserved for patients whose intraocular pressure has not responded to drops or trabeculectomy. Once again this is carried out under a local anaesthetic, administered via an injection placed either behind the eye or under the surface of the eye. This procedure needs to be carried out in an operating theatre but can be done as a day case. It takes about 10 minutes and may make the eye ache for a few hours afterwards. Anti-inflammatory and antibiotic drops and painkillers are administered after the procedure. Diode laser treatment works by applying energy to the ciliary body, thereby damaging the process by which the aqueous fluid is produced and reducing the intraocular pressure. Although it is extremely effective in reducing pressure, the ciliary body often repairs itself and the pressure rises once again, requiring repeat diode laser treatment. Sometimes four or five treatments may be required.

Combined trabeculectomy and cataract surgery

If you have glaucoma that is not satisfactorily controlled with drops and you also have cataracts, the eye surgeon may recommend that you have an operation that combines cataract surgery with trabeculectomy. This is a well-recognised procedure and, enables you to have the benefit of the trabeculectomy and the cataract surgery in one operation. The operation takes slightly longer than trabeculectomy alone and can take up to an hour. Once again this can be carried out under a local or a general anaesthetic (see below).

BENEFITS AND RISK OF SURGERY FOR GLAUCOMA

Any form of surgery carries a small risk and should be carried out only after the benefits of the surgery have been carefully weighed against the potential risks. You should discuss with your eye specialist the indications for surgical treatment, its benefits and risks. Trabeculectomy is

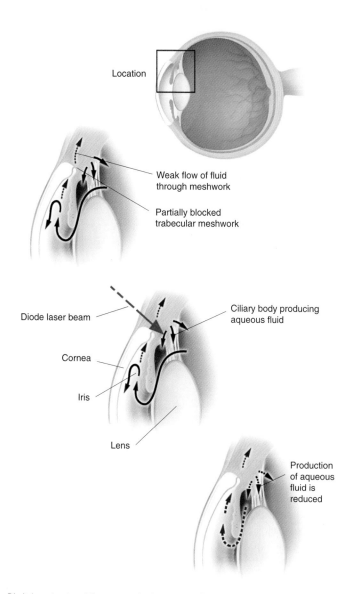

Location

Weak flow of fluid
through meshwork

Partially blocked
trabecular meshwork

Diode laser beam

Cornea

Iris

Lens

Ciliary body producing
aqueous fluid

Production
of aqueous
fluid is
reduced

Diode laser treatment for open-angle glaucoma works by applying laser energy to the
ciliary body, thereby damaging the process by which the aqueous fluid is produced and
reducing intraocular pressure.

QUESTIONS TO ASK YOUR CONSULTANT

1. What benefits should the surgery provide?
2. What are the risks if surgery isn't performed?
3. How many of these procedures have you carried out? With what results?
4. What are the possible risks and complications?
5. How long will I need to stay in hospital?
6. How long will it take my eye to heal?
7. Will my vision improve significantly?
8. Are there any activities that I should avoid afterwards?
9. Will I need ongoing medication?
10. Will I need a change of spectacles after the operation?

usually highly beneficial and successfully controls the intraocular pressure in the great majority of cases. The treatment is often so successful that the eyedrops that have been used previously to control the pressure can be stopped. The side effects of trabeculectomy include bleeding within the eye at the time of surgery (hyphaema), but this usually clears readily after a few days although it can blur the vision in the meantime. Another potential side effect occurs when the drainage bleb is too effective and drains the fluid out of the eye too quickly, thereby making the eye softer than it should be. Once again this is usually self-limiting and the problem resolves as the operation heals. Surgery for open-angle glaucoma can predispose to the development of a cataract in the eyes, although this is usually readily operated upon and dealt with by cataract surgery (see above).

Over the first few years there is an increasing risk that the trabeculectomy bleb ('water blister') can heal over and stop functioning, although often the operation can successfully reduce the pressure in the eye for life. This premature healing of the bleb is particularly prevalent in patients of African origin or in people below the age of 40. Under these circumstances the surgeon may opt to use special drops (an antimetabolite) during surgery which reduce the risk of premature healing, but can sometimes lead to over-draining of the bleb. Infection of the eye (endophthalmitis) is a rare complication of trabeculectomy. If the bleb heals over and stops functioning, it can be opened up again by the surgeon using a simple procedure under local anaesthetic ('needling') – see page 68.

ASSESSMENT BEFORE THE OPERATION

This is similar to that required for cataract surgery (see page 37), apart from the fact that measurements of the length of the eye (biometry) are not necessary. The eyes will be examined before the operation to check that there are no potential sources of infection such as conjunctivitis and blepharitis (infection of the lids), which would be treated with antibiotics before surgery would be considered. Equally any source of infection elsewhere in the body such as a urinary infection or leg ulcer would also need to be treated. It is important to let your eye surgeon know if you believe you have any of these potential sources of infection.

THE ANAESTHETIC

For a trabeculectomy or combined trabeculectomy and cataract surgery, a local or general anaesthetic is required and is identical to the anaesthetic used in cataract surgery (see page 42).

POSTOPERATIVE RECOVERY AND TREATMENT

Most people have a pad put on the eye for a few hours after the operation and when this is removed the vision may be initially quite blurred. The vision should gradually improve over the first post-operative week but new spectacles may well be required and you should go to your optometrist/ optician approximately one month after the surgery as advised by your eye surgeon.

The eye surgeon will probably want to see you the day after the operation and then again at approximately one week and four weeks after the operation. During this period your eye will be treated with antibiotic and steroid or other anti-inflammatory drops, but you will not need to continue with the glaucoma drops for the eye that has been operated upon. The glaucoma drops will, however, be necessary for the other eye if it has not had surgery, and you need to seek the advice of the eye surgeon about this point. The eye may ache a little after the operation but this is usually satisfactorily controlled with a mild oral analgesic in combination with the prescribed drops. Recovery of the eye is otherwise similar to that after cataract surgery (see page 43) and most people can return to work after approximately two weeks. Once again heavy lifting and straining need to be avoided for the first six weeks after surgery as this can cause a rise in pressure in the eye which can potentially damage the wound.

If all is well at the time of the one-month postoperative appointment, the surgeon will probably return to the previous pattern of monitoring the glaucoma as an outpatient two to three times a year.

As mentioned above, over the years the bleb formed during trabeculectomy can gradually heal over. If this does occur the trabeculectomy can be repeated or sometimes your eye surgeon will carry out a simple 'needling' procedure. This involves inserting a needle into the bleb and breaking down the scar tissue to allow the bleb to function satisfactorily once again. This is also carried out under a local anaesthetic and can be carried out either as an outpatient procedure or sometimes as a day case in the operating theatre. This procedure is simple and more straightforward than the original trabeculectomy operation.

KEY POINTS

✓ Surgery for glaucoma (trabeculectomy) is usually straightforward and has good results

✓ Serious complications are rare

✓ Laser treatment is also available but is usually reserved for those cases where drainage surgery (trabeculectomy) has already been tried

✓ After successful glaucoma surgery, the glaucoma treatment drops can usually be discontinued for the operated eye, but will need to be continued in the other eye if this has not had surgery

✓ After surgery the glaucoma still needs to be monitored with outpatient appointments two to three times a year

Macular degeneration

Macular degeneration is the most common cause of poor eyesight in people aged over 60. It never leads to complete sight loss, because it is only the central vision that is affected. However, in most cases, it is difficult or impossible to treat.

WHAT IS MACULAR DEGENERATION?

Macular degeneration is an eye condition that affects the central (reading) part of the vision. It is caused by disease changes at the most highly developed part of the retina, the macula, which is made up of millions of light-sensitive cone and rod cells. The macula is situated at the centre of your retina at the point where most of the light rays coming into the eye are focused. It is responsible for the central vision and for detailed visual activities, such as reading and writing and the ability to appreciate colour. In macular degeneration the highly specialised cells at the macula stop functioning, either partially or completely. Macular degeneration usually affects both eyes, although it tends to be asymmetrical affecting one eye more than the other.

TYPES OF MACULAR DEGENERATION

Age-related macular degeneration is by far the most common form of macular disease and affects about 500,000 people in the UK. It mostly affects people aged over 60 and is more common with increasing age. Other conditions such as macular dystrophies (see later) are much rarer and tend to affect younger people.

Age-related macular degeneration

Age-related macular degeneration is loosely divided into two main types: the 'dry form' and the 'wet

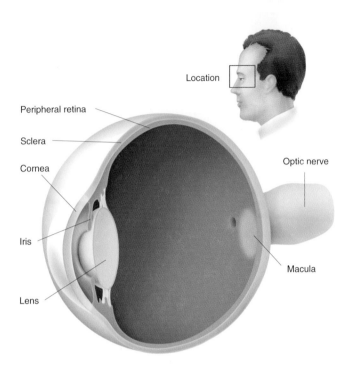

Location

Peripheral retina

Sclera

Cornea

Optic nerve

Iris

Macula

Lens

Macular degeneration is caused by disease changes at the most highly developed part of the retina, the macula, which is made up of millions of light-sensitive cone and rod cells.

form'. The dry form, which cannot be treated, tends to be slow in onset. It is caused by a gradual failure of the delicate cells that control the central vision at the macula. It is more common than the wet form of the disease and is not associated with water logging or haemorrhage at the macula – hence the description of the condition as 'dry'.

In dry age-related macular degeneration, important supporting cells of the retina (retinal pigment epithelial cells/RPE cells) start to malfunction and die and can lead to patches of atrophy (like a worn carpet) interspersed by pigment clumping with a characteristic appearance. As the retinal pigment epithelial cells die off there is an associated loss of the retinal receptor cells (the rods and cones), thus resulting in a reduction in the function of macular vision.

The wet variety (seen in less

than 20 per cent of cases) can have a much more rapid effect on the eyesight, sometimes causing a severe loss of central vision within a matter of days. It is caused by the growth of abnormal blood vessels through age-related defects in the deepest layer of the retina (usually in the macular region). These abnormal vessels form a membrane that is called a 'choroidal neovascular membrane'. They can leak, causing water logging of the macula and affecting central vision. In addition, they are fragile and can bleed, causing scarring. The wet variety of macular degeneration is also known as a 'disciform maculopathy' or a 'subretinal neovascular membrane'. It can occasionally be treated with laser therapy which ablates the blood vessels and closes them off (see page 75).

The precise cause of age-related macular degeneration is unknown. It is thought to be related to the genetic 'clock' of the specialist macular cells, which start functioning abnormally and eventually die. The dry form of the condition usually occurs before the wet variety and both frequently coexist, although the wet variety is less common.

Age-related changes at the macula are often seen in eyes of people over the age of 60. These changes are commonly seen in people with normal vision and do not always lead to the degenerative changes of the macula that reduce sight. The most common age-related finding at the macula consists of yellowish-white spots in the retina called 'drusen'. These represent an accumulation of the by-products of the metabolism of the retina in the deepest layer of the retina (Bruch's membrane) and are associated with a failure of the retinal pigment epithelial cells. Drusen are divided into two varieties according to their appearance: 'soft drusen' which are round and less distinct than the other variety, and 'hard drusen', which have a glinting appearance. Drusen alone do not affect visual function, but may presage the development of dry or wet macular degeneration as described above. This is more likely with soft rather than hard drusen. The detailed diagnosis of this condition is specialised and requires an examination by a hospital eye specialist.

Age-related macular degeneration may also be more common in some families, although a precise pattern of inheritance has not been determined and most cases have no family history. Smoking has been identified as a predisposing factor and all people at risk from macular degeneration should not smoke. There has also been some evidence that deficiencies in vitamins A, C and E, and the trace metal zinc, contribute to the cause of macular degeneration.

Macular dystrophies

Macular dystrophies are much rarer than age-related macular degeneration and often affect people at a younger age. They develop when the specialist cells in the macula stop working normally. Many macular dystrophies are inherited or congenital and in these forms it is believed that this malfunction is the result of defects in the genetic make-up of the cells.

Other causes of macular disease

Trauma (usually involving a direct blow to the eye) can cause damage to the macula and lead to macular degenerative changes at the time or later in life.

Some medications have been linked to macular damage, but usually only in very high doses. These include antidepressants (such as chlorpromazine), drugs used in the prevention and treatment of malaria (such as chloroquine), tamoxifen (used in the treatment of some breast cancers) and some medicines used to treat rheumatoid arthritis (hydroxychloroquine and chloroquine). If you are worried about whether your medicines can cause or worsen macular degeneration, you should read the information leaflet provided with them. If this leaflet suggests macular degeneration and/or damage to the macula as a potential side effect, you should seek advice from your GP or hospital eye specialist.

Short-sightedness (myopia) can predispose to the development of macular degeneration, which usually comes on later in life but can occur at a younger age than 'age-related' macular degeneration. The precise mechanism for this is not fully understood.

AGE-RELATED MACULAR DEGENERATION

Who is affected?

Age-related macular degeneration becomes increasingly common as people become older. Many people have signs of ageing (see page 71) at the macula but retain good vision. Both men and women are affected equally and there do not appear to be any particular differences between races or geographical origin. Age-related macular degeneration can coexist with cataracts and/or glaucoma, but these conditions do not predispose to the development of macular disease.

Symptoms

In the early stages, you may notice that images are blurred or distorted (for example, straight lines may look kinked) and that there is a change in the size of the image, with objects looking smaller or larger than with the other eye. You may also find that reading becomes difficult and that you miss out letters or words.

If only one eye is affected, you may not notice these early symptoms. However, later on, the vision may be further affected so that there appears to be a blank spot or dark patch in the centre of the sight, faces are difficult to recognise and reading is even more difficult. Driving may not be possible. Some people with macular degeneration notice a dark patch in the centre of their vision when they wake in the morning, but find that this patch gradually fades over about half an hour. The appreciation of colour may be affected, although this may not be noticable. The eyes may be sensitive to bright light and, if the condition is advanced, flashes of light or unusual images may be seen. The detailed central vision may be particularly affected in conditions of low lighting. Although the central vision may eventually be lost, people with macular degeneration alone never lose their eyesight completely because the peripheral (side) vision is always retained. This means that almost everyone with macular degeneration will have enough vision to get about without any help and can maintain their independence.

If you notice a sudden onset of any of the above symptoms, particularly distortion in your central vision, you should seek urgent advice from your optometrist and/or GP, who will refer you to an eye consultant or the eye accident and emergency department as necessary. A sudden onset of symptoms can sometimes indicate the beginnings of the wet variety of macular degeneration, which can, very occasionally, be treated with a laser.

Diagnosis

Macular degenerative changes may first be noted by the optometrist and/or your GP during a routine eye examination and can occur before any of the associated symptoms arise. If these changes are significant and/or you are experiencing symptoms, you will usually be referred to a hospital eye consultant to confirm the diagnosis.

This usually involves a comprehensive examination of the eye, including the dilation (widening) of the pupils with drops to give a better view of your retina. It should be noted that these drops blur the vision and preclude driving for six to eight hours afterwards, so drivers should arrange alternative transport home.

If the wet form of macular degeneration is suspected, a fundus fluorescein angiogram (FFA) may be performed (see figure below). This involves injecting a fluorescent dye (fluorescein) into a vein in the arm and taking a series of colour photographs of the retina as the dye passes through the blood vessels in the back of the eye. These photographs give an accurate map of the changes occurring at the macula, and help the eye specialist to decide whether you have the 'dry' or 'wet' form of the disease, and whether laser treatment is possible.

The angiogram usually takes less than 10 minutes to perform. It is not painful, but may make you feel light-headed or a little nauseous,

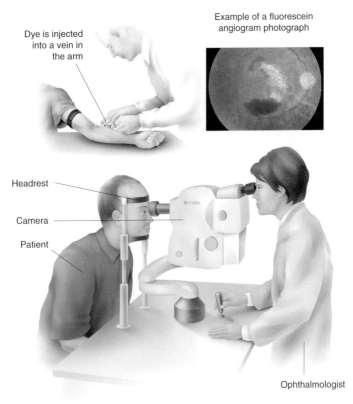

Dye is injected into a vein in the arm

Example of a fluorescein angiogram photograph

Headrest

Camera

Patient

Ophthalmologist

A fundus fluorescein angiogram (FFA) can be used to study the blood vessels at the back of the eye. A fluorescent dye is injected into the arm, and a series of photographs taken as the dye flows through the blood vessels in the back of the eye.

and the light from the camera can be quite dazzling for a few minutes afterwards. The dye used for the injection causes a transient yellow discoloration of the skin, and turns the urine yellow as it is excreted from the body over the next 24 hours.

Treatment

For the dry form of macular degeneration, there is usually no medical treatment. It has been suggested that dietary supplements of vitamins A, C and E, and zinc may be helpful but this is theoretical and has not been the subject of scientific trials. More recently there has been some evidence to support treatment with a dietary carotenoid called lutein which is available commercially as a nasal spray and tablet. It is known that lutein is present in large quantities in the normal macular tissue, and is readily available in the diet, particularly in red and green peppers, sweetcorn, spinach and eggs.

For the wet variety, argon (thermal) laser treatment can occasionally delay the progression of the disease but is appropriate only in a small number of cases (about ten per cent). If the subretinal membrane of vessels (choroidal neovascular membrane) impinges on or is very near to the very central part of the macula (the fovea), treatment with argon laser to the membrane will usually destroy the central vision and is therefore of no benefit. If the membrane is situated away from the fovea, argon laser treatment can be used to ablate and close down the blood vessels in the offending membrane. In these cases, the treatment is successful in about half the patients, but unfortunately there is a 50 per cent chance of recurrence within three years. Laser treatment tends to lead to dying off (atrophy) of the overlying retina in the region of the treatment, and this may be noticed by the patient as a blank patch in the vision.

Laser treatment is carried out as an outpatient procedure and involves the pupil of the affected eye being dilated with drops. Local anaesthetic drops are then applied and a contact lens placed on the eye. As the local anaesthetic numbs the eye, the contact lens is not felt and keeps the eye open so that you do not need to be concerned about blinking. The laser treatment is then applied with the patient sitting at the slit-lamp biomicroscope (similar to that used to examine the eye). The flashes of laser light are very bright and can lead to the eye being dazzled for half an hour or so after the procedure. Laser treatment of this kind is not painful. It is probably helpful to ask a friend or relative to accompany you to the hospital for laser treatment and you should not drive until the effects of the dilating drops have worn off (six to eight hours), and then only if your vision is good enough. People who have the wet form of macular degeneration should discuss the possibility of treatment with their hospital eye specialist.

Various optical aids are available for people with poor vision caused by macular degeneration and these are described below under the section entitled 'Aids for those with poor vision' (see page 84).

Monitoring macular degeneration

The dry form of macular degeneration usually progresses gradually and the eyesight is never lost completely as peripheral vision is retained. It is possible to monitor the condition by assessing changes in the symptoms, especially the reading vision. More formal monitoring of distance and reading vision can be done by the optometrist and/or eye specialist who can also chart the changes in the retina. However, regular monitoring by the hospital eye specialist is not normally required.

A special chart is available from the eye consultant to help you monitor your eyesight (an Amsler chart). An example is shown opposite together with instructions for its use. The chart is particularly helpful in recognising the onset of

distortion in the central vision. To use it, you need to wear reading spectacles and test each eye separately (with your other eye covered with the palm of your hand). The Amsler chart consists of a black central spot surrounded by a grid of horizontal and vertical black lines. You should concentrate on the central black spot and see whether any of the grid lines are distorted or any part of the image on the chart is missing.

Getting help

If you believe that you have macular degeneration or are at risk of developing the disease because of a positive family history, you should first visit your optometrist for a check-up, explaining your concerns and symptoms. If your optometrist believes that you have significant macular disease (or your symptoms persist), you should consult your GP (your optometrist can refer you to the GP), who will arrange an appointment with the hospital eye specialist if necessary.

Sometimes, patients with known wet macular degeneration in one eye are advised to phone their hospital eye accident and emergency department as soon as possible if they get a sudden onset of symptoms in their previously unaffected eye. You should discuss this with your hospital eye specialist.

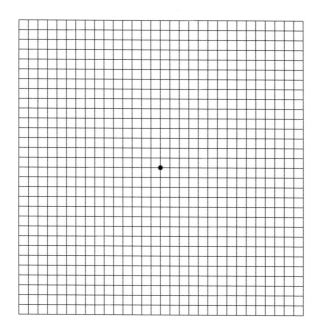

An Amsler chart can help you monitor your eyesight.

Instructions for use

1. Place this page at eye level and where light is consistent and without glare.
2. Put on your reading glasses and cover one eye.
3. Fix your gaze on the centre black dot.
4. Keeping your gaze fixed, try to see if any lines are distorted or missing.
5. Mark the defect on the chart.
6. TEST EACH EYE SEPARATELY.
7. If the distortion is new or has worsened, arrange to see your ophthalmologist urgently.
8. *Always* keep the Amsler chart the *same distance* from your eyes each time you test.

DRIVING AND MACULAR DEGENERATION

If the vision is affected by macular degeneration, driving may become more difficult particularly at night or in conditions of poor light. There are strict regulations laid down by law and administered by the Driver and Vehicle Licensing Agency (DVLA) at Swansea. The vision does not need to have deteriorated very greatly to fail to achieve the legal visual requirements for driving and, if you have doubts, you should visit your local optometrist for a check-up and advice.

Many people with mild macular degeneration are able to drive normally, although some choose not to drive at night or when the lighting conditions are poor.

If you are advised that your vision does not meet the legal requirements for driving, you should inform the DVLA at Swansea. It should be noted that motor vehicle insurance is not valid if the driver's vision falls below the legal standard.

RECENT ADVANCES IN AGE-RELATED MACULAR DEGENERATION

Over the past few years, there has been a lot of interest and research in the treatment of age-related macular degeneration. Although there has been no significant progress in preventing the onset of the disease, there are a number of medical trials in progress concentrating on the treatment of the wet form of the disease. These potential new treatments are outlined below.

Photodynamic therapy (PDT)

This is used to treat the wet form (exudative or neovascular disease) in which a membrane of fragile new blood vessels grows beneath the retina. The treatment is appropriate only for certain cases of wet macular degeneration (your hospital eye specialist can advise you about this) and has no place in established damage from wet macular degeneration or in the dry variety. The treatment uses a cold laser beam (low energy), which does not damage normal retinal tissue. This contrasts with the high-energy, thermal, argon laser therapy conventionally used to treat disciform maculopathy.

Before treatment with the cold laser, a substance that is sensitive to light (photosensitive) is injected into a vein in the arm. This substance is derived from a group of naturally occurring compounds called 'porphyrins'. It concentrates in the abnormal blood vessels at the macula by attaching to the vessel walls, allowing the energy from the laser to be targeted at the abnormal vascular membrane, thereby destroying it. Although the vascular membrane regresses after the laser treatment, there is evidence that it tends to regrow within the first six months and to require further treatment. Repeated treatment can cause retinal thinning and loss of the specialist cells in the macula, mimicking the dry form of macular degeneration.

It should be emphasised that photodynamic therapy cannot restore sight to a macula with established retinal damage. Treatment with photodynamic therapy is currently being evaluated in clinical trials on both sides of the Atlantic and much more work is required before definitive advice can be given about its effectiveness. At the moment it is not routinely available as a treatment within the NHS.

Radiotherapy

Low-dose radiotherapy to the subretinal neovascular membrane has also been the subject of extensive research in recent years and, although initial results were encouraging, it appears that the treatment damages the overlying retina as well as the affected membrane. Further evaluation is required before this form of treatment can be recommended.

Other treatments

Retinal translocation has excited considerable press interest, but is in the early stages of development and is appropriate only for a very small number of patients with the wet form of macular degeneration. It involves moving the retinal tissue away from the underlying membrane before treating the membrane with a laser, therefore avoiding damage from the laser to the overlying retina. Once again, this is not available as a routine NHS treatment and its efficacy is still being evaluated.

There is also some experimental work being carried out in animals involving the transplantation of parts of the retina, but the work is at a very early stage. In the distant future, gene therapy may be possible for people with a family history of the disease but, as a specific gene for age-related macular degeneration has yet to be identified, this form of potential therapy remains purely theoretical.

Finally, it cannot be overemphasised that people with macular degeneration alone will never go blind or lose their sight completely. If people with macular degeneration have been registered as partially sighted or blind, this simply means that their central vision has deteriorated to a very low level.

Cataracts can often be present at the same time as macular degeneration and if these develop it may well be worth having cataract surgery in order to improve the vision. For more details, see page 32. Your hospital eye consultant can advise you about this.

KEY POINTS

✓ The most common form of macular degeneration is age-related and affects people over the age of 60

✓ There are two main forms of age-related macular degeneration: 'wet' and 'dry'

✓ People with macular degeneration alone never lose their sight completely and will always retain their peripheral (navigational) vision

✓ There is no treatment for most forms of macular degeneration, but low vision aids (see next section) can help the sight

Registration as blind or partially sighted

If you have very poor central vision and/or significant loss of visual field in both eyes, you can be registered as partially sighted or blind; this will enable you to obtain help and support from your local Social Services Department. Registration can be arranged only by a hospital eye consultant who, after examining your eyes, will complete the necessary paper work and forward this to your local Social Services Department for the Visually Impaired. The Social Services Officer will then get in touch with you and will usually arrange a home visit to discuss placing you on the appropriate register and to talk about available help such as help at home, improved lighting and various home gadgets for people with poor sight.

As well as the benefits outlined in the box on pages 82–3, you may be entitled to the Attendance Allowance (if you are over 65 years of age), Invalid Care Allowance, Invalidity Benefit, Severe Disablement Allowance (SDA), Disability Living Allowance and/or Disability Working Allowance. For further information, contact your local Social Security Department, Citizens Advice Bureau (CAB), Welfare Rights Officer or Specialist Social Workers at the Social Services Department.

You can also look at the Royal National Institute of the Blind's leaflet on free prescriptions and the Wales Council for the Blind's leaflet on disability. For contact details, please see Useful addresses, page 86.

BENEFITS OF REGISTERING AS BLIND OR PARTIALLY SIGHTED

	Registered blind	Registered partially sighted
• Special personal income tax allowance	Yes	No

Apply to local Tax Office – proof of registration may be required.

• Additional Income Support Benefit (Disability Premium)	Yes	No

Apply to your local Benefit Agency.

• Exemption from 'Non-dependants' deductions from Income Support	Yes	No

• Additional Housing Benefit	Yes	Yes

Proof of Registration will be required when applying to the local housing department.

• Exemption from 'Non-dependants' deductions	Yes	Possible

• Exemption from Council Tax	No	No

• TV licence at reduced cost	Yes	No

Registered blind people are entitled to an annual reduction. A certificate will be issued by your local Social Services Department for you to take to the post office when you renew your licence.

• Postage concessions	Yes	Yes

Applies to certain articles including braille material and spoken recordings, such as Talking Books and Talking Newspapers, but not personal tapes or typed letters. Details are available from the Royal National Institute of the Blind.

	Registered blind	Registered partially sighted
• Telephones	Yes	Yes

Financial assistance by the Social Services Department towards the cost of installing a telephone may be given in cases that meet the criteria for the Chronically Sick and Disabled Persons Act 1970. Applications are subject to an assessment of need.

• Telephones for the Blind Fund	Yes	No

This is a national charity that may give financial assistance in some cases. Apply to your local Social Services Department, where your application will be assessed against the criteria laid down by the Telephones for the Blind Fund.

• Bus passes	Yes	No

These are available to any person over the age of 16 years who is registered blind. Apply to your local Social Services Department.

• Disabled Person's Car Badges	Yes	Yes

If you are registered blind you may apply for a Disabled Person's Car Badge. Application forms are available from your local Social Services Department. People who are partially sighted may be eligible if they have an additional disability.

• Disabled Person's Railcard	Yes	Yes

Application forms are available from your local post office, and British Rail Travel Services.

• Free eye test	Yes	Yes

National Health Service (NHS) Eye Examination Fee.

Aids for those with poor vision

There are many practical aids that can be helpful to those with poor vision. These include talking watches, talking clocks, large dial telephones and timepieces. Advice as to where these can be found in your locality can be obtained from the specialist social workers at the local Social Services Department. Guide dogs can be immensely helpful and advice regarding the appropriateness and eligibility for a guide dog can be obtained from the Royal National Institute of the Blind (RNIB) – see Useful addresses, page 87.

Spectacles

If you have macular degeneration, you should ensure that your spectacles are checked annually by your optometrist. This will ensure that you are getting the most out of your vision.

Low vision aids

These consist of very strong spectacles (magnifying spectacles) and telescopes that enlarge the image to allow it to fall on the part of the retina not affected by the macular degenerative process. If a very large area of the retina is affected, these low vision aids are usually not helpful. The hospital eye specialist can refer those who would benefit from a trial of these aids to a specialist optometrist either in the community or in the hospital. Low vision aids are available free through the NHS although private assessments are also possible.

Closed circuit television systems (CCTV) may be of help in some circumstances. These consist of a video camera that will photograph a piece of text, magnify it and project it on to a screen. These systems are expensive and can cost up to £2,000; they are seldom available on the NHS. Once again advice about their availability can be obtained during a low vision aid assessment. The information may also be available through the local branch of the RNIB.

Books and newspapers

Large print books are available from all libraries and through most good book shops. Talking newspapers and talking books are also obtainable – more details are given in Useful addresses, page 86.

Lighting

Good bright lighting is essential to get the best out of your vision. An anglepoise or standard lamp with a strong bulb is helpful for reading, sewing and close work. Halogen bulbs create a good light without the heat that accompanies conventional light bulbs. Good daylight is helpful, so many people read in front of a sunny window.

KEY POINTS

✓ If you have very poor central vision, you may be entitled to register as partially sighted or blind

✓ Visual aids, audio books and magazines are available for people with poor vision

✓ Good lighting can help people with poor vision to read and do close work more easily

Useful adresses

Calibre Cassette Library
New Road, Weston Turville
Aylesbury
Bucks HP22 5XQ
Tel: 01296 432339
Fax: 01296 392599
Email: enquiries@calibre.org.uk
Website: www.calibre.org.uk

Library of 6,000 titles of unabridged books on standard cassettes. Proof of disability allows borrowing for membership in return for voluntary donations.

Guide Dogs for the Blind Association
Hillfields
Burghfield
Reading RG7 3YG
Tel: 01189 385555
Fax: 01189 835433
Email: guidedogs@guidedogs.org.uk
Helpline: 0870 600 2323
Website: www.guidedogs.org.uk

Provides guide dogs, mobility and other rehabilitation services to enable blind and partially sighted people to lead the fullest and most independent lives possible.

Health Development Agency
Trevelyan House
30 Great Peter Street
London SW1P 2HW
Helpline: 0800 555777
Website: www.hda-online.org.uk

Formerly Health Education Authority; now only deals with research. Publications on health matters can be ordered via helpline.

Look, National Federation of Families with Visually Impaired Children
c/o Queen Alexandra College
49 Court Oak Road
Harborne
Birmingham B17 9TF
Tel: 0121 428 5038
Fax: 0121 427 9800
Email: office@look-uk.org
Website: www.look-uk.org

Offers information, help and support for parents who have visually impaired children; access to benefits, education and grants. Runs youth project for young people aged 9–18 years.

Macular Disease Society
PO Box 16
Denbigh LL16 5ZA
Tel: 01745 816212
Fax: 01745 812179
Email: maculardisease@hotmail.com
Helpline: 0800 328 2849
Website: www.maculardisease.org

Provides information, a regular magazine *Side View*, and practical support for people with any of the eye conditions covered by the term macular disease. Promotes research into macular disease.

National Association for the Education, Training and Support of Blind and Partially Sighted People (OPSIS)
Court Oak Road
Harborne
Birmingham B17 9TG
Tel: 0121 428 5037
Fax: 0121 428 5048
Email: opsis@dircon.co.uk
Website: www.opsis.org.uk

Association of independent charities working together to provide services for visually impaired people.

Partially Sighted Society
PO Box 322, Doncaster
S. Yorkshire DN1 2XA
Tel: 01302 323132
Fax: 01302 368998
Email: info@partsight.org.uk

Assists visually impaired people to make the best use of their remaining vision with a range of useful publications and equipment available by mail order.

Royal College of Ophthalmologists
17 Cornwall Terrace
London NW1 4QW
Tel: 020 7935 0702
Fax: 020 7935 9838
Website: www.rcophth.ac.uk

Professional college for eye specialists who produce a number of leaflets in conjunction with the Royal National Institute of the Blind about a variety of eye diseases.

RNIB Talking Books Service
PO Box 173
Peterborough PE2 6WS
Tel: 020 7388 1266
Fax: 01733 375001
Email: cservices@rnib.org.uk
Helpline: 0845 702 3153

For annual membership fee (£57 in 2002) offer loan of machine and talking books.

Royal National Institute of the Blind (RNIB)
105 Judd Street
London WC1H 9NE
Tel: 020 7388 1266
Fax: 020 7388 2034
Email: rnib@rnib.org.uk
Helpline: 0845 766 9999
Website: www.rnib.org.uk

Offers a range of information and advice on lifestyle changes and employment for people facing loss of sight. Also offers support and training in braille. Has mail-order catalogue of useful aids.

Royal National Institute of the Blind, Cymru

Trident Court, East Moors Road
Cardiff CF24 5TD
Tel: 029 2045 0440
Fax: 029 2044 9550
Email: stuart.davies@rnib.org.uk
Helpline: 0845 766 9999
Website: www.rnib.org.uk

Offers a range of information and advice on lifestyle changes and employment for people facing loss of sight. Also offers support and training in braille. Has mail-order catalogue of useful aids.

Sense Cymru

5 Raleigh Walk
Brigantine Place
Cardiff CF10 4LN
Tel: 029 2045 7641
Fax: 029 2049 9644
Email: enquiries@sensecymru.fsnet.co.uk
Website: www.sense.org.uk

Offers information, advice and support to people who are deaf–blind as a result of rubella and have associated disabilities. Can refer for assessment as appropriate.

Talking Newspaper Association UK

National Recording Centre
Browning Road
Heathfield, E. Sussex TN21 8DB
Tel: 01435 866102
Fax: 01435 865422
Email: info@tnauk.org.uk
Website: www.tnauk.org.uk

List 200 national newspapers and magazines on tape, computer, CD-ROM and email for loan to visually impaired, blind and physically disabled people.

Wales Council for the Blind

3rd Floor
Shand House
20 Newport Road
Cardiff CF2 1YB
Tel: 029 2047 3954
Fax: 029 2043 3920
Email: staff@wcbnet.freeserve.co.uk
Website: www.wcb-ccd.org.co.uk

Charity umbrella body for visually impaired organisations and local authorities in Wales. Information on benefits and general welfare as well as training for professionals and technological advice for visually impaired people. Transcription service.

THE INTERNET AS A SOURCE OF FURTHER INFORMATION

After reading this book, you may feel that you would like further information on the subject. One source is the internet and there are a great many websites with useful information about medical disorders, related charities and support groups. Some websites, however, have unhelpful and inaccurate information. Many are sponsored by commercial organisations or raise revenue by advertising, but nevertheless aim to provide impartial and trustworthy health information. Others may be reputable but you should be aware that they may be biased in their recommendations. Remember that treatment advertised on international websites may not be available in the UK.

Unless you know the address of the specific website that you want to visit (for example, familydoctor.co.uk), you may find the following guidelines helpful when searching the internet.

There are several different sorts of websites that you can use to look for information, the main ones being search engines, directories and portals.

Search engines and directories

There are many search engines and directories that all use different algorithms (procedures for computation) to return different results when you do a search. Search engines use computer programs called spiders, which crawl the web on a daily basis to search individual pages within a site and then queue them ready for listing in their database.

Directories, however, consider a site as a whole and use the description and information that was provided with the site when it was submitted to the directory to decide whether a site matches the searcher's needs. For both there is little or no selection in terms of quality of information, although

engines and directories do try to impose rules about decency and content. Popular search engines in the UK include:

google.co.uk
aol.co.uk
msn.co.uk
lycos.co.uk
hotbot.co.uk
overture.com
ask.co.uk
espotting.com
looksmart.co.uk
alltheweb.com
uk.altavista.com

The two biggest directories are:

yahoo.com
dmoz.org

Portals

Portals are doorways to the internet that provide links to useful sites, news and other services, and may also provide search engine services (such as msn.co.uk). Many portals charge for putting their clients' sites high up in your list of search results. The quality of the websites listed depends on the selection criteria used in compiling the portal, although portals focused on a specific group, such as medical information portals, may have more rigorous inclusion criteria than other searchable websites. Examples of medical portals can be found at:

nhsdirect.nhs.uk
patient.co.uk

Links to many British medical charities will be found at the Association of Medical Research Charities (www.amrc.org.uk) and Charity Choice (www.charitychoice.co.uk).

Search phrases

Be specific when entering a search phrase. Searching for information on 'cancer' could give astrological information as well as medical: 'lung cancer' would be a better choice. Either use the engine's advanced search feature and ask for the exact phrase, or put the phrase in quotes – 'lung cancer' – as this will link the words. Adding 'uk' to your search phrase will bring up mainly British websites, so a good search would be 'lung cancer' uk (don't include uk within the quotes).

Always remember that the internet is international and unregulated. Although it holds a wealth of invaluable information, individual websites may be biased, out of date or just plain wrong. Family Doctor Publications accepts no responsibility for the content of links published in their series.

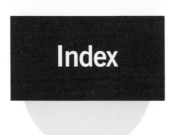

Index